Women and Fibromyalgia

Women and Fibromyalgia

♦

Living with an Invisible Dis-ease

Barbara A. Keddy, RN, Ph.D.

iUniverse, Inc.

New York Lincoln Shanghai

Women and Fibromyalgia
Living with an Invisible Dis-ease

iUniverse books may be ordered through booksellers or by contacting:

iUniverse
2021 Pine Lake Road, Suite 100
Lincoln, NE 68512
www.iuniverse.com
1-800-Authors (1-800-288-4677)

Because of the dynamic nature of the Internet, any Web addresses or links contained in this book may have changed since publication and may no longer be valid.

ISBN: 978-0-595-44371-0 (pbk)
ISBN: 978-0-595-88700-2 (ebk)

Printed in the United States of America

The information, ideas, and suggestions in this book are not intended as a substitute for professional medical advice. Before following any suggestions contained in this book, you should consult your personal physician. Neither the author nor the publisher shall be liable or responsible for any loss or damage allegedly arising as a consequence of your use or application of any information or suggestions in this book.

Contents

Acknowledgements ix

Foreword. xi

Introduction xv

CHAPTER 1   The Fibromyalgia Syndrome 1

CHAPTER 2   Meet the Women 27

CHAPTER 3   Pain, Fatigue, Sleeplessness, and Often
             Depression. 46

CHAPTER 4   Women and Fibromyalgia 57

CHAPTER 5   Triggers, Attacks, and Supports: Women
             Speak Out 68

CHAPTER 6   Treatments But No Cure: What Can Be Done? 77

CHAPTER 7   Midlife, Menopause, and Fibromyalgia 86

CHAPTER 8   Women Spirit 94

CHAPTER 9   Disability: Struggling To Be Believed/Struggling
             For Economic Security 102

CHAPTER 10   Words of Wisdom from Wise Women 121

CHAPTER 11   Women Revisited 127

Notes 133

Fibromyalgia Resource List 153

Bibliography 165

Acknowledgements

Unless a person actually lives with someone in constant pain accompanied by a myriad of other physical ailments, it is impossible for him or her to know the extent of emotional and physical support that may need to be provided day after day. Not everyone with fibromyalgia is as fortunate as I have been to have had a caregiver as loving and patient as my life partner, Milton. Without him, I would not have been able to live life to the fullest in spite of the many challenges of living with my demon called fibromyalgia. This book would not have been possible without him.

The women in this book show me what it is like to live with courage in the face of the many obstacles they experience every waking day. To them I owe a debt of gratitude.

Professionals such as massage therapists and chiropractors who are engaged in body work have made life much more manageable for me. In particular, I am thankful to Peter Goodman, Dr. Dena Churchill, and Jackie Blackburn for the many hours, over many years, in which they have provided body work to relieve my pain, giving me relief in times of great distress. Mind and body work cannot be separated, and they have provided relief for both.

Thank you to my children, my sister Nancy, my cousin-in-law Jack, and my friend Marty for listening to me complain about pain over and over again, year after year, and always providing patient, listening ears.

To all the sufferers of fibromyalgia, chronic fatigue, and environmental illnesses, I acknowledge your struggles and hope that some day these so-called *invisible* conditions will be considered worthy of becoming more socially and politically *visible*.

It is Dr. Roy Fox at the Nova Scotia Environmental Centre who led me to the conclusions I made in this book, and to him I express my gratitude. Dr. Stewart Cameron and Dr. Robert Stalker are physicians who have provided kindness and compassion as well as excellent medical advice for many years. I am grateful for their sensitivity and understanding about fibromyalgia. Dr. Stalker read a first draft of the book and graciously provided feedback.

There are many friends who have supported me through difficult times. The list seems endless. It is sufficient to say that without these relationships I would not have been able to have had such a full and happy life in spite of living with fibromyalgia as my unwanted companion. I wish that all of you who also have these daily challenges could have the love that comes from such friendships to help guide you through each day.

Finally, thank you Adam Chew for your patience in guiding me through the process of setting up a web site. I am indeed technologically challenged. Michael Fiedler at iUniverse deserves a medal for putting up with my whining and constant questions. He did so with charm and grace. I am eternally grateful.

Foreword

It is devilish to suffer from a pain that is all but nameless. Blessed are they who are stricken only with classifiable diseases! Blessed are the poor, the sick, the crossed in love, for at least other people know what is the matter with them and will listen to their belly-achings with sympathy.

—George Orwell, *Burmese Days*

The description of fibromyalgia as a clinical syndrome can be outlined in medical prose, always succinct and terse in textbooks. It is a common, chronic musculoskeletal condition characterized by widespread chronic pain, specific tender points, sleep disturbance, and chronic fatigue. There are many other symptoms that commonly accompany the disorder, including migraine and tension-type headaches, Raynaud's syndrome, irritable bowel syndrome, and fleeting numbness. The American College of Rheumatology (1990) has set the diagnostic criteria. There are no pathognomonic tests. It occurs nine times more in women than men, and it can occur at any age but mostly between ages thirty-five to fifty. Its cause is unknown, but one third of all cases have some relationship to trauma. Academic discussions follow about the factors that may play a causal role: social and psychological influences; frustrating and unfulfilled life situations; un-restorative sleep, neurochemical and metabolic factors; abnormal brain responses and neural plasticity; and substance P and gate-control mechanisms of pain in the nervous system.

What the textbook approach to medical conditions does not capture are the experiences of the person who suffers and the attitudes of physicians and others who see no abnormalities on x-ray, no specific lab-test abnormality, and no obvious physical defect. Dr. Keddy captures the patient's experience of living and coping with suffering in the poignant interviews with twenty women who have fibromyalgia, herself included.

In recent years, there has been more attention to the need to hear the voice of the person with an illness. Knowing what gene defect produces Huntington's chorea does not help us understand the suffering and pain of a mother worrying about the fate of her children. Knowing the classification of Hodgkin's disease does not help us understand the experience of going through repeated chemotherapy in the way artist Robert Pope showed us in his ninety-four paintings of the experience of illness before he died of his disease.

Fibromyalgia is a common disorder affecting many people, mostly women, and we need to hear their voices to understand what this condition does to them and their lives. In this book, we hear of their strengths, their weaknesses, their frustrations, their ways of effectively coping, and the ways they just can't manage. We also hear of the supports they receive and the lack of understanding shown by many who don't believe their suffering is real. We hear of physicians who don't believe in things they can't test and measure and of others who do provide understanding and support.

When people suffer, they will seek relief. And if relief is not there, they will seek an explanation. When physicians cannot offer relief and don't understand the situation well enough to explain, the sufferer will seek solace elsewhere. It is sobering but not surprising that almost all twenty women interviewed by Dr. Keddy seek relief from alternative medicine and alternative therapists.

It is not difficult to conclude that fibromyalgia is a major medical and social issue of concern to physicians, employers, workers' compensation boards, the courts, the insurance industry, and ultimately society, but during all of the discussion and wrangling we must take time to hear the voices of those who suffer. Today we demand evidence-based medicine to bring convincing data for each statement and conclusion, but there is still an important place for what people believe and what people feel.

In this book, we will hear the voices of twenty women—what they believe and what they feel.

Pain ... cannot recollect
When it begun—or if there were
A time when it was not—
It has no future—but itself ...

—Emily Dickinson, Poem 650

Dr. Jock Murray
OC, MD, FRCP(C), MACP, LLD(HON), DSc (HON), FRCP(LON)

Introduction

"How *can* you keep working?" she asked me a few seconds after we had introduced ourselves. As that interview proceeded, I knew I would write this book as an account of my journey through pain, fatigue, and sleeplessness and to illustrate how I was able to keep on working when so many others living with the fibromyalgia syndrome (FMS) could not. I would share women's stories of living, suffering, and struggling with FMS and highlight women's courage while living with this unbelievably common, debilitating, and chronic condition. This is not a book just for scholars and health professionals, and it is not strictly about FMS. Rather, it is for anyone interested in the mind/body connection and the psychosocial implications of being a woman in contemporary society. My storytelling allows voices that have until now been mostly silenced to be heard.

An integral part of this book is the midlife women who so kindly took the time to share their experiences. They gave me the incentive to keep going as I painfully sat for hours at my computer. I knew some of these women personally before undertaking this project; others were new to me. As they shared cups of tea and coffee with me, willingly recounting story after story of their struggles, we immediately recognized the ties that we shared as FMS sufferers. If one of us stretched in her chair or stood up after sitting for awhile, the other smiled knowingly. One woman said she recognized the "fibromyalgia sitting-to-standing awkwardness" and noted she had even identified it once in a stranger on a train. Equally as obvious to our group was the recognizable body position that we, as fibromyalgia pain sufferers, adopt when walking down stairs.

Although the twenty women in this book (one of whom is me) have different life histories, the fibromyalgia syndrome and its symptoms are common to us all. In spite of our class and race differences, we all shared one experience: as black or white women, we had all lived lives highly attuned to our environments since childhood.[1]

By sharing our stories, the invisibility of the difficulties we experience on a day-to-day basis are made visible in spite of our contrasts in economic privilege, colour, relationships with others, ethnicity, age, and other pre-existing medical conditions such as chronic fatigue, environmental sensitivities, and even multiple sclerosis. We are united in our struggles to understand why these things are happening to our bodies and what was to follow next.

I interviewed most of the women in person only, but I combined face-to-face interviews and e-mail communication with some. The women came from various parts of Canada from the east coast to the west. If we twenty women from diverse backgrounds experience the same phenomena, it is probable that most other women with FMS also share our experiences. In fact, research from around the world supports this claim. I will refer to a number of these studies in upcoming chapters.

Most surprising during the year-and-a-half interview process was how much we all knew about this demon known as fibromyalgia. I believe I have lived with it the longest of the women I interviewed, although I did not have an official diagnosis until almost three decades after my symptoms began. However, even the newly diagnosed women knew so much more than I had during my long journey toward understanding this condition. By the time a physician actually said there was little doubt that I had FMS, I already knew it. I did not join a support group; I did not just want a discussion with strangers on the Internet; and I did not want scientific descriptions about all the physiological aspects of FMS that affect muscles and nerves. I wanted to have control over my body and to make my own decisions about how I would live with what I perceived to be a life sentence. I could not believe that there is no cure. (However, I have learned that there are remissions from acute attacks, and there are things I can do sometimes to help myself stave off acute attacks and to acknowledge the relationship of mind and body.)

What I wanted from this research was face-to-face contact with sufferers so I could find common themes that would allow me to make my own educated guess about a possible cause. What I wanted was this book—a book that validates my experiences and offers me hope that I can take back control of my body despite the pain, fatigue, and sleeplessness that will probably never go completely away. I did not really expect answers to the longstanding, puzzling questions about FMS, particularly after years of extensive research literature on the topic.

Nevertheless, I did experience an epiphany as a result of the shared dialogue with these women. I lived through an "aha" moment that led me to a possible—and, to my way of thinking, a likely—explanation of the gendered nature of FMS, a mystery that has plagued researchers since the condition was named. The result of this extraordinary moment is the journey I make in this book while writing about FMS and *why* I believe it is a syndrome that strikes mostly women, an issue that is not discussed nor theorized about elsewhere.

Many books intended for those who suffer from fibromyalgia, chronic fatigue, and chemical sensitivities tend to focus primarily on how to live with the conditions. While there is value in that approach, I believe we need more answers about why these conditions occur and, most importantly, why they are more common in women. I hope I will give my readers some food for thought as I take a different path toward understanding the nature of FMS in particular, even though there are many similarities among the three conditions. Specifically, I want to explore the relationship between women and FMS and the political, psychosocial determinants of health that I believe are precursors to its occurrence. Many of the chronic conditions that women with FMS endure, including depression, must be analyzed within a socio-political context.

I have long been aware that until relatively recently women's health has been sorely neglected by the scientific community. When women need health care, they are often viewed as the sum parts of their reproductive capacity. Researchers have been slow to explore diseases and conditions that are more common to women than men or are not directly related to reproduction. Of late, I have noticed the willingness of women to speak to the neglect they feel when principally defined as premenstrual, menstrual, child bearing, peri-menopausal, menopausal, or postmenopausal, while serious conditions that primarily affect women, like the common fibromyalgia, are often obscured.

This book is about women who suffer from what has been defined as a mysterious, invisible, or, worse, nonexistent condition. As such, it is a validation of genuine pain and suffering. It is based upon my years of research about FMS and my own lived experiences. Throughout the book as I present the literature on FMS, I will also share my own current and past experiences and my thoughts as I relate to the issues; these thoughts and experiences will be presented in italics. While the stylistic practice of endnotes can be somewhat frustrating to the reader, I believe that they have made for a smoother flow of the reading. These endnotes are somewhat lengthy but hopefully add to the valuable information contained therein.

In chapter 1, I will explore current theories, symptoms, medical and complementary treatments, and policy implications. I will present the latest available data regarding theories, characteristics of the condition, and possible causes and explain why I use the term "syndrome" rather than "disease." The commonalities in symptoms between fibromyalgia, chronic fatigue syndrome (CFS), environmental illness (also known as multiple chemical sensitivities, or MCS), and, more recently, Gulf War syndrome will also be briefly discussed in this chapter. I will then venture to speculate about what I believe to be the cause of FMS, which to this point has not been articulated or discussed in the literature. It is this personal theory that will guide the rest of this book. A relatively brief summary of relevant neuroanatomy will be presented in order to augment my proposed theory. I deliberately present this information before introducing the women I interviewed. As one who has reflected extensively on their narratives, reviewed the literature in great depth, and lived the experience of an FMS sufferer, I hope I have written a theoretical treatise that will bring together the various components of the issues regarding causation and place the common symptoms of FMS within the context of the syndrome.

In chapter 2, I will introduce the readers to the women in the research study. A short description of our lives, ages, and professional and personal life histories will be an engaging way to understand the courage it takes to face each day when living with a chronic condition. To protect confidentiality, I will not reveal their real names or geographic locales. Each of the women defines what FMS means to her. These specific views will be presented briefly in this chapter and further explored in following chapters as their narratives continue.

In chapter 3, the women describe what it is like to live with pain, fatigue, loss of sleep, and depression on a day-to-day basis. The "lookin' good and feelin' bad" characteristics of FMS will come alive as we listen to their voices. The ways in which our experiences are similar and different will be explored.

Chapter 4 of this book poses a theory that the commonalities in the personalities of the women can shed light on why FMS is more common in women than in men. I will postulate that *women* with FMS have unique and similar ways of "being" in the world, which can precipitate the condition.[2] While I explore this issue, I also emphasize that it is dangerous to stereotype a woman with FMS as having a certain personality type because there are ramifications if the condition becomes "psychologized." Nonetheless, I believe this issue is crucial to understanding FMS. In spite of the inherent dangers of stereotyping, readers may be surprised at the commonalities among the women.

Can flare-ups and remissions be controlled? What precipitates an acute episode? What kinds of supports are needed in these times? Are relationships a help or a hindrance? What is it like to live with an invisible condition? Is it really an illness?[3] Knowing that others cannot see our pain, we may live with guilt, depression, fear, disappointment, anger, and the label "hypochondriac." These are the main foci of chapter 5 as the women describe emotions and experiences that guide their everyday lives. Since I am not alienated from most of the experiences and emotions, I will use the collective pronouns "we" and "our" throughout the book.

"What can be done?" is the question I ask in chapter 6. I find some of the answers from the women themselves, as well as from others who have reported their experiences in the literature. How do we live with this condition, which strikes arbitrarily without warning in acute episodes and lays in wait with dull pains, fatigue, and other symptoms on a consistent, somewhat permanent basis? I will present the various mechanisms from allopathic Western medical approaches to the complementary practices that the women and I have used in dealing with FMS. How many of us became our own medical advocates and investigators and the experts of our own lives is a key issue in this chapter. How a marginalized group of women identify themselves against a dominant group of medical practitioners will be briefly explored. I will elaborate upon my own experiences regarding what has been helpful to me.

Since most of the women I spoke with were in midlife, I will focus on menopause and FMS in chapter 7. I am interested in women and aging and how the psychic power of ageism impacts on our lives. Is the "brain fog," or lack of concentration, that FMS sufferers speak of the result of menopause, aging in general, FMS, or even something related to women's ways of living in a patriarchy? These are the questions I will pose to the readers.

Chapter 8 is called simply "Women Spirit." It is the chapter in which I outline the power of midlife women to transcend obstacles in spite of the effort it takes. The "keep on movin' along" approach to life is one of courage, which most women have while tackling FMS and trying to find peace and relief from symptoms. Who is in charge: the FMS or the women? The issues are complex, yet they are simultaneously intriguing and frustrating.

The economic and psychological costs of FMS within a society that does not recognize "invisible" health conditions are tremendous.[3] Policy implications, particularly regarding long-term disability, are the focus of chapter 9. Employers are generally unhappy with this diagnosis, and physicians are in a bind as health-care providers struggle to appease insurance companies while treating their patients. FMS is perceived by some to be of epidemic proportions, and if this is so, then third-party payers are faced with growing concerns about insurance payments. For that reason, physicians are often hesitant to even name the diagnosis as FMS, resulting in even more angst for those who suffer from this debilitating condition. Constructing health histories is a tedious process, but one that many women face in order to have their stories taken seriously.

Older women, the "crones" whose advice has for so long been ignored, speak up in the next chapter of this book. Here, advice is freely given from some of the women who know how to access the system and take control of their own bodies. Chapter 10 emphasizes a move from the negative to the positive in the hope that the readers may be inspired by these stories of courage and optimism to make change in their own lives or the lives of their loved ones. It is about beating back that demon and taking back control of our lives and our bodies. It is also a chapter about what could be done by women whose own needs take second place to those of others.

Finally, a brief final chapter will inform the readers about ten of the women five years later and the paths that their lives have taken since the initial interviews.

The purpose of this book is not to generalize the experiences of twenty women to all women who have fibromyalgia. It is a study with a variety of research participants telling their stories, and the end result is the development of a theory about why this condition occurs and why it occurs more commonly in women. As with all theories, it is meant to be tested with scientific rigor and cannot be said to represent absolute truth. Nonetheless, the stories do represent different women from diverse backgrounds. Their similar experiences have led me to the analysis I present in the chapters to follow.

It will be obvious that this book will steer away from a critique of a purely mechanistic scientific/medical paradigm in favour of one that takes into account lived experiences and an intuitive understanding of a body/ mind connection in fibromyalgia. The reductionist view is based upon research based on clinical drug trials, the study of genetic factors, the search for abnormalities in muscles and brain patterns with regard to sleep and pain, speculation about growth hormone defects, and bone density issues as well as other biomedical etiologies. None of this research has resulted in a cure for this syndrome. Health professionals basically attempt to *treat* the symptoms. I do not mean to imply that this kind of research is useless. In fact, relief from these symptoms is what all of us seek with great fervour.

However, recent claims of intended pharmaceutical trials searching for a cure for fibromyalgia is, in my view, misleading, as I do not believe that drugs to cure this condition are possible. Nonetheless, there is a juxtaposition based upon our Western desire to find a cure for what ails us without pause for reflection regarding psycho-social structures that are detrimental to our health. I cannot say with certainty that there is or is not a biomedical cause for FMS. What I hope to do is broaden our understanding of the interconnectedness, rather than the duality, of the two paradigms.

This is a book which should interest all those who have fibromyalgia, generally accompanied by chronic fatigue, and often chemical sensitivities, their families, and researchers who are interested in this myriad of conditions. Academics and researchers who are involved with women and health will also find the issues thought-provoking and informative, but—even more significant—this book will propose a theory of causation that can be tested by others. I grappled with the difficulty of writing a book that tries to marry everyday people who live with FMS and health professionals and researchers who are anxious to explore the "why" question, and this continues to be somewhat problematic. I do not, however, succumb to talking down to those who are suffering, and for that reason I provide more medical information than might be needed.

I do not venture into the arena of very serious, immediate life threatening allergies, like that of someone allergic to peanuts or penicillin, for example. An allergy is more *immediately* serious than that of a chemical sensitivity (referred to as Multiple Chemical Sensitivities or Environmental Illness). MCS/EI can occur with or without fibromyalgia and chronic fatigue. By MCS/EI I mean recurrent symptoms to many or some chemical compounds. This does not mean however, that chemical sensitivities cannot develop into more serious allergies or that they do not affect quality of life issues. Unfortunately the term is one which is hotly debated and sometimes negatively referred to as a 20th Century phenomenon by those who do not believe in its existence. The distinction between an allergy and a chemical sensitivity is often confusing.

To summarize, we are at a crossroads regarding the understanding of FMS and hopefully this book will shed new light on the condition or provide another link in the unravelling of this mysterious ailment.

1

The Fibromyalgia Syndrome

The attempt to describe fibromyalgia is usually reduced to a recitation of the most common symptoms. Pain, usually described as "sore all over" or general stiffness; non-restorative sleep, often referred to as "twilight sleep;" often overwhelming fatigue; and depression are among the most commonly cited symptoms that physicians hear. These are often combined with a host of many others, including sensitivities to environmental chemicals, bowel and digestive upsets, headaches, lack of concentration (sometimes referred to as "brain fog"), and muscle cramping. Singly, together, or in various configurations, these symptoms make up what can currently best be described as fibromyalgia syndrome (FMS).[1] They do not in and of themselves make up a specific disease entity, a theory regarding etiology, or a description of cause and effect. Although it is called a disease by some, particularly those who believe it to be a form of arthritis, I will consistently refer to fibromyalgia as a syndrome, because it is more a set of symptoms than a disease that is even minimally understood.

The term "syndrome" is used to describe a condition that has a set of consistent symptoms but, unlike a disease, has no proven cause. Although many have speculated about whether or not FMS begins as a result of an injury, a surgery, a virus, chemical exposure, or psychological trauma, no cause can be stated with certainty. Consequently, the search for symptoms becomes integral to the disease model in an effort to legitimate the actual condition.

FMS is difficult to diagnose, because the only test for its presence is based upon pain in pressure sites, of which there are said to be eighteen paired points on either side of the body. If a person experiences pain upon applying pressure to at least eleven of these paired points, and there is a history of widespread pain for at least three months, then a diagnosis of FMS can be made.[1] The usual kinds of laboratory tests do not reveal abnormalities, therefore pressure-point testing is often considered to be a rather unscientific and nebulous method of diagnosis by those who would prefer more technological and scientific rigor.

It is difficult to ascertain which of the main descriptors just mentioned begin before the others, or if they occur simultaneously. It is the old chicken and egg dilemma. Is concentration difficult because of lack of sleep? Is a person depressed because many activities are curtailed or because of the presence of pain or because of lack of sleep? Does the struggle with pain cause the fatigue? Does the fatigue go hand in hand with depression? Even more perplexing is whether or not all chronic pain is actually FMS. How to unravel these mysteries has been a daunting task for many. It is little wonder that the primary medical focus has been on attempts to treat symptoms rather than on causality, while the scientific research has explored such things as the physiology of muscles and brain patterns that influence sleep and pain in those with the condition. Although there are several theories regarding cause, they are highly speculative and controversial and, in fact, many believe FMS exists only in the person's imagination. For those of us with this agonizing condition, we can say with certainty that the pain is not imagined.

FMS has been called malingering by many. According to Kerr, since 1998 in the United States, "When your MD attends his [sic] continuing medical education courses, fibromyalgia is being described as 'simple aches and pains.'"[2] In my experience, this is no longer quite accurate, as many of the younger, and some older family physicians, seem to know something about and try to be more accepting of FMS as a real, not imagined, condition. However, this condition is often not easily recognized or diagnosed as a complex set of symptoms that together make up a specific syndrome, and many sufferers spend years searching for answers. Misdiagnosis is responsible for loss of work, sleeplessness, chronic suffering from pain, family stress, depression, guilt, and low self-esteem, and unfortunately it often takes months, if not years, before the condition is properly diagnosed.

The prevalence of fibromyalgia is debatable; some speculate that as many as ten million people are affected in North America, while other numbers vary from 2 percent to 3 percent of the population. These estimates are no doubt unreliable because many sufferers go undiagnosed, and it is therefore difficult to obtain exact numbers. We do know that fibromyalgia affects primarily women. The reason for this is not known.

Women and Fibromyalgia

While this book is not intended to criticize physicians, other health professionals, or researchers for their lack of understanding about FMS, it is necessary to point out that women's health in general has been sadly neglected or misrepresented. It follows, therefore, that a condition which affects primarily women and is difficult to diagnose and treat would frustrate most health-care professionals. Fibromyalgia continues to be the invisible disability about which little is known regarding etiology, but the lived experience of those who spend each day with the symptoms and who try to find ways to alleviate some of them or try to be taken seriously is evidence of the disabling life sentence. Leon Chaitow[1] refers to those with fibromyalgia as the "walking wounded" and the "vertically ill." For the women who continue to try to find answers while dealing with the day-to-day stress entailed in their daily activities, it can become almost an overwhelming existence, particularly if the women have jobs inside and outside the home.

It is often pain that most plagues the person suffering from FMS, yet women often minimize the verbal expression of pain. Pain itself is essentially a gender issue since it is widely known that men and women present different ailments with different language to their doctors. A man reporting chronic pain is generally treated more seriously than a woman. A woman's complaints are often denied, minimized, or attributed to her imagination. The dissonance in the discourse of pain reporting between men and women results in different types of responses from the medical profession and it is women who are disadvantaged.[3]

Similarly, most medical research is also gender biased, taking for granted the male as norm. For example, leaders of the now classic, decades-old aspirin study with 25,000 men assumed that the findings could be extrapolated to women and concluded that it was advisable for women as well as men to take a daily dose of aspirin to avoid cardiovascular problems. Yet in October 2003, Harvard University researcher Eva Schernhammer found abnormalities among women who take aspirin. While following 88,000 nurses for eighteen years, she and her team discovered that the incidence of pancreatic cancer in women increased significantly for those who took acetylsalicylic acid regularly. It is understandable that researchers would prefer that their research subjects (laboratory animals or humans) were male since their hormonal fluctuations are easier to control for than those of women. However, that does not excuse the scientific community from the neglect and errors that have been committed in the past with regard to women's health. Even worse has been the negligence with regard to women's propensity to certain conditions.

Is it probable then that, because it is more frequently seen in women, FMS is less likely to be as thoroughly investigated than if it were more common in men? Why are women's voices appropriated so frequently in spite of reported sufferings?

"These aches and pains are part of growing older. After all, you're menopausal. What can you expect?" the resident doctor asked me many years ago. Who believes me? I am a woman with an invisible disability! I look healthy but feel absolutely awful most of the time, particularly when the pain is so intense. Pain is my constant companion.

While little has been known about women's health in general until the past two decades, why FMS is more common in women is a perplexing issue. It is possible that FMS episodes can be precipitated by occupational hazards, yet it is rarely regarded as work related in spite of the frequency of missed work days and the many female workers who are on long-term disability or workers' compensation with this condition in certain occupations. Stress in the workplace accompanied by repetitive motions that are common among female clerical workers, muscular-skeletal injuries because of constant lifting done by those in factories and the service industry or nursing, or work done by women in the home are generally not thought to be contributors to the problems in the first place. In fact, I could speculate that FMS could also be precipitated by such normal biological changes as menstruation, childbirth, or menopause.

While these possibilities are themselves rarely explored in great depth as gendered potential causes of fibromyalgia, I believe there are other more serious structural and psycho-social reasons for its prevalence among women, which are even more complex than the purely psychological common view that women have a dysfunctional response to stress. This perspective lends credence to the myth of the hysterical female psyche. There are probably multiple truths to causation of FMS, and the issue of prevalence among women remains one of the most challenging.

Just how much more prevalent FMS is to women than men is controversial; the ratio estimates vary from 4:1 to 10:1.[4] Nevertheless, it is a serious women's health concern. Women visit doctor's offices for the multiple symptoms, chiropractors, physiotherapists, massage therapists, and acupuncturists for pain more frequently than men, and women report more environmental/chemical sensitivities and illnesses than their male counterparts. What can be done? Who listens to women's voices?

"Since you're postmenopausal you will never have the body you had before, so aches and pains are to be expected; it's nothing serious," says the young medical resident. I feel like I am swimming against the tide. There aren't any answers. This pain is just not the normal aches and pains of aging; it is incapacitating. The fatigue is debilitating.

Theories and Speculations

There are more questions than answers regarding a theoretical understanding of FMS. In fact, the debate among physicians, and especially among rheumatologists, is even controversial. It is interesting to note that FMS has been called the second-highest ranking arthritis disorder in Canada.[5] Presumably it came to be associated with arthritis because FMS involves multiple muscle aches and pains. The word itself is a combination of the Latin roots "fibro" (connective tissue fibers), "my" (muscle), "al" (pain), and "gia" (condition of).[6] The degree of reported prevalence seems to be a major concern of many physicians, particularly because of the consequences of diagnosing people who will have difficulties with long-term disability, workers' compensation, and other third payer insurance benefits. For these reasons, fibromyalgia is a political issue that has the medical profession unprepared for the challenges of diagnosing.

Two Canadian physicians, White and Harth, point out that FMS "is a syndrome of unknown pathogenesis without known specific laboratory markers."[7] In their 1998 critique in the *Journal of Rheumatology* of an article by Wolfe and his colleagues,[8] they discuss how difficult it is to have accurate statistics about the prevalence of FMS. They criticize Wolfe for saying that FMS "is out of control." They ask how he arrived at his conclusion that 2 percent of the adult population has FMS. In fact, reported numbers of people affected vary considerably.[9] It is indeed very difficult to estimate the prevalence of FMS since so many who suffer from this debilitating yet invisible syndrome do not report it out of fear of being labelled hypochondriacs or because they are unable to find physicians who are willing or knowledgeable enough to present the patient with the diagnosis. The debate among rheumatologists is ongoing and controversial but is rarely as dramatic as the ensuing letters to the editor about "The Fibromyalgia *Problem*," (my italics) following Wolfe and Hadler's articles[10] in a prestigious journal. All of this shows that because there is a lack of scientific knowledge (defined as that which can be quantified or show cause and effect) regarding etiology, the many similar symptoms of all FMS sufferers is somehow the fault of those who experience them. While there are many conditions for which there are no known definite causes, FMS is treated less as a serious, debilitating disorder than one that is more visible and easier to diagnose. This is true in spite of the fact that there are serious consequences for those who suffer from this debilitating condition, and it is especially true when people are worried about not being believed.

I am sitting with a group of women, all of them nurses, discussing environmental illness and the fact that one Canadian claimant recently lost a case in court. "Do you really believe that all people who say they have environmental illness, chronic fatigue, fibromyalgia really have it? Is there even such a thing?" asked one nurse.

I experience that same disquiet that I do when I am faced with disbelievers. "Does she think I make up FMS?" I think to myself. But, I keep quiet. In fact, I rarely discuss this condition with anyone! To do so is to risk ridicule. I live with pain sometimes so extreme that I have to cry out. I am indeed walking wounded, but I walk quietly.

Devon Starlanyl, a medical doctor, has written extensively about FMS. She believes that it has finally "come out of the closet" and that it has been known and described since the early 1800s by William Balfour, a surgeon in Scotland in 1815. She describes the various names under which it has been known: rheumatism, myalgia, and fibrositis. Wallace and Wallace also give an extensive history of this long-ago noted condition.[11] In an article in *Alternative Treatments for Fibromyalgia and Chronic Fatigue Syndrome*, Starlanyl writes that myofascial pain (a localized, painful musculoskeletal condition) is often confused with FMS.[12] She points out that people can have both, but that the pain of FMS is generalized while that of myofascial pain is more regional. However, often one can have both conditions and go undiagnosed. This can lead to extreme frustration as the sufferer frequents more and more doctors, all unable to find specific causes for the pain.

One is left to wonder if our forebears who complained generally of rheumatism were not actually suffering from FMS, myofascial pain, or polymyalgia, which also resembles these conditions and is an inflammation of the large muscles of the body. The Arthritis Foundation calls FMS "soft tissue rheumatism."

I asked the resident physician: "What is wrong with my wrist? It hurts so much, and it's sometimes swollen. See? Here."

"Oh, you must have sprained it sometime," he said while giving it a cursory examination.

"It has been that way off and on for three years and aches constantly!" I tell him. I give up mentioning it to any medical practitioner even though my wrist seems worse under certain conditions. I wonder if it is soft tissue rheumatism, a fancy word for fibromyalgia. It seems to be triggered by barometric changes. Now I never mention my fibromyalgia to a physician.

Types, Characteristics, and Possible Causes of FMS

Types

There are various speculations about the kinds of FMS. Romano postulates there are three: (1) idiopathic or primary FMS, which occurs for unknown reasons as a result of such things as stress or weather changes; (2) secondary FMS which occurs with people who have well-recognized, chronic medical conditions (such as two of the women in this book who also have multiple sclerosis); and (3) posttraumatic FMS, the result of an accident or trauma.[4]

"I can't understand why I can't walk. My knees hurt. I feel sick all over. I have pain everywhere, and my legs won't work. All of this following a long labor and C section, but how can the doctors think I have gout? I'm only twenty-five! You'd think they could find out what is happening to me," I recall thinking after the birth of my first child.

Khraishi[13] believes that nearly half of the people with FMS have developed it following an injury or accident, while the rest have not had a definite injury. Khraishi is careful to note that while there are many theories regarding causes, there are none that are conclusive.

Characteristics

In the *Canadian Journal of CME,* Khraishi[13] writes that the incidence of FMS peaks between the ages of twenty-five and forty-five years, while

Chaitow[1] believes that FMS pain increases with age. In my personal experience, it has increased with age.

While Khraishi believes that FMS peaks in younger years, there is even more confusion regarding its onset. Soderberg, Lundman, and Norberg from Sweden believe that it afflicts mostly middle-aged women.[14]

Not only do the prevalence, ratio of women to men, the onset, and possible causes vary from country to country and researcher to researcher, but Meisler[15] believes there are inconsistencies in the data regarding the prevalence of specific areas of pain, such as back and chest pain. He postulates that pain attacks one area of the body more frequently than another depending upon the person's age. I have not read about this theory anywhere else, but I believe his view warrants attention, as do most of the researchers who attempt to make sense of what is, to this point, a very mysterious and confusing syndrome. However, none of the above-mentioned researchers address why this occurs primarily in women; rather they speculate about the characteristics of the syndrome.

Causes

Khraishi is careful to note that while there are many theories regarding causes, there are none that are conclusive. The links between FMS and chronic fatigue syndrome raise the possibility that it could be infectious, but he maintains that this is not yet substantiated.

There are those who argue that the cause of FMS may be genetic and hereditary in terms of predisposition, and there are also many who believe that the end result, that is the pain associated with FMS, is key to understanding what happens chemically to the muscles of FMS sufferers. It is thought that only then can effective treatment occur. Among those are the ones who believe that the pain is caused by malic acid and magnesium deficiency.[16]

Does cal/mag help? I have this restless leg symptom that is common in fibromyalgia. I think that's secondary, but most practitioners suggest that cal/mag deficiency is the cause. On a Web site with Florence Cardinal, I learned there are two different kinds of restless legs, one with pain and the other without. I learned more from Web sites than from any health-care provider about this syndrome. But the jury is still out on whether or not malic acid and magnesium can help pain in the legs or elsewhere.

Some endocrinologists suggest that there is a decreased nocturnal level of prolactin and growth hormone in women with FMS.[17] There are others who believe there is a genetic link.[18] Still others searching for the biological etiology are convinced that FMS is due to inadequate thyroid regulation of tissues,[19] another debate among endocrinologists. The search for a medical cause continues, but the focus is on tissues and cells and on the muscular-skeletal, endocrine, or nervous systems that have been affected. It appears to me that this is putting the cart before the horse. These may be the physiological effects, but what is the cause?

Conversely, there are many who believe that there are psychological and/or biopsychosocial inadequacies, for whatever reasons, within the population of people with FMS.[20]

Finally, there are the views of the complementary and/or alternative practitioners who do not ascribe often to the usual allopathic treatments or scientific paradigm but rather speculate about causation and reach conclusions with less rigorous methods—but often with more interesting results. Sahley, for example, reports on a study in the *Journal of Nutritional Medicine* in which fifteen patients were given an oral magnesium and malic acid preparation; within forty-eight hours, all reported significant pain relief.[16] Most naturopaths and homeopaths are familiar with a nutritionally based approach as a means of relief but not as a cure. Still, dosage, body weight, gender, menopausal, ethnic, and racial differences are not used as a basis for prescribing these preparations, and this makes for a less-than-accurate or untrustworthy approach.

In addition to inconsistencies in prescribing these alternative or complementary medicines, there are other difficulties. Those who do not believe in homeopathy suggest that it is simply a placebo from a kindly practitioner who helps the client deal with the trauma of fibromyalgia. Just as allopathic medicines are not adjusted for certain physiological characteristics of individuals, herbal or homeopathic concoctions are also not regulated for differences in body types. There is also the issue of expense. Vitamins, supplements, and homeopathic preparations are not covered by medical insurance. For the economically deprived and women already overburdened with attempts to find relief from painful and aggravating symptoms, the costs of supplements are often prohibitive.

I have tried homeopathic drops and various herbs. They have not helped. I do take several vitamins and supplements, which are very expensive. What do others do who cannot afford them? While I am not sure they actually help, I do have a hunch that the immune system is boosted by them. This is a serious social-class issue, as only the privileged few can afford to take these regularly and in such high doses. I asked a homeopathic practitioner who is also a medical doctor about the causes of FMS from his point of view. He said "genetic predisposition, chemical exposure, and abused victim personality." These are issues I do pay great heed to, but I hesitate to use the words "abused victim personality." That sounds like blaming the woman and re-victimizing her! Yet, I know he did not mean it in that particular way. Furthermore, I don't know if it is a genetic predisposition. Early socialization about trying to meet another person's needs and sensing with heightened acuity what those needs are, resulting in a lifetime of over-stimulating the nervous system, seems a more likely answer. But I give away too much too soon of the theory I am postulating.

In summary, there are those who believe that FMS might be caused by genetics, viruses, body systems disorders, nutritional deficiencies, or psychological factors. In my view, all of those factors may be interrelated, but I do not believe that any one of them in isolation is entirely responsible for causing fibromyalgia. Instead, I have reached the point whereby I am eager to present my own theory. I believe that FMS is a neurological disorder or, more specifically, a psycho-neurological condition brought about by oppressive social structures within society. In an unusual twist, I am presenting a theory running fast ahead of the evidence, which I believe will follow in subsequent chapters.

My Theory: Psycho-Neurological Overload

While I claim a specific theoretical framework as my postulate, which guides my thinking about the cause or predisposition to FMS, I cannot say that this theory is entirely of my own making. I build instead on the work of others who have led me to this path. I believe there is a particular personality type that is prone to FMS. This individual is what Elaine Aron calls the "highly sensitive person," Forssen, Carlstedt, and Mortberg describe as "compulsive sensitivity," and Roger Easterbrooks calls the "ultrasensitive person."[21] Women have generally been the gender most responsible for the affective needs of others; this is crucial to my belief about why FMS affects women in such large numbers. However, I do not think that personality type alone, described strictly as a woman's identity, can precipitate FMS, as not all extremely sensitive persons have fibromyalgia and not all women are prone to an exaggerated sensitivity. Therefore, it is likely that there are other factors—such as an accident, extreme or continuing anxiety, surgery, or even posttraumatic stress—which combined with this specific personality result in this painful condition. These are complex issues and difficult to unravel. Furthermore, there are inherent dangers in suggesting such an idea, which can result in stereotyping of women. In fact, FMS should not be framed as strictly a woman's malaise as it does also affect men and some children.

Do I believe that it is hereditary? I do not know if it is genetic or socially induced as a result of being parented and socialized in a certain mode (which brings up the nature/nurture issue). I do believe that for FMS to develop certain precursors in addition to a susceptible personality (which I have come to believe is that of a compulsively sensitive, or highly sensitive, or ultra-sensitive person) must be in place:

• A chronic or acute illness

• An injury

• An environmental toxin

- A prolonged or dramatic psychological stress that the autonomic nervous system (ANS) of the highly/ultra-sensitive person (CS/HSP/USP) can no longer tolerate

These may gradually over-stimulate the nervous system or build until an acute attack is initiated by something in the environment or by stress that the autonomic nervous system can no longer endure.

Since the 1960s there has been a great deal of attention to the role of women in society. Women are generally more aware than men of the emotional and physical needs of others. They have a tendency to anticipate the responses of others to social circumstances and to attend to perceived needs. When this awareness of others becomes *super* heightened, then there is the sense of always being "on duty." In my view, it is even more than that. I believe that fibromyalgia is a heightened ability to see and feel emotions of others—to know, or actually feel if someone is happy, afraid, stressed, or anxiously in need of care. I go on at the risk of sounding too new age. I believe that the person with fibromyalgia experiences something like an aura in the presence of others, which results in energy becoming "stuck" within her own nervous system—energy that cannot be released as she tries to deal with all these perceived needs of others. This energy clings to an overloaded nervous system that is constantly in a state of arousal or disharmony. Eastern practitioners of health could perhaps liken this to chi (Qi) being stuck and resulting in physical problems such as insomnia, depression, anxiety, chemical sensitivities, body pain, and, of course, fibromyalgia.

It is theorists such as Elaine Aron[21] who have inspired me to believe that highly sensitive people are prone to FMS. While Aron elaborates on the term highly sensitive person (HSP), she does not make or intend to make a link between HSP and ailments or diseases such as fibromyalgia. However, I was struck by her definition of an HSP, as it is congruent with how the women in this book define themselves. In my view, the woman who develops FMS is someone who believes that her life role is to better the lives of others first, to the exclusion of her own needs, and she does this by being highly attuned to her environment more so than most women.

While men may also take on that role, males are generally not socialized the same as females, and societal expectations are usually not the same.

But personality type aside (in fact, I would argue that it is not a personality trait but rather an inability to learn how to switch off intense reactions to the emotions of others), there is little doubt that other kinds of conditions must be present before FMS develops. I am interested in how, eventually, even environmental factors such as weather conditions, particularly barometric changes, and their effects on an HSP can precipitate an acute episode, bringing more pressure to bear on the autonomic nervous system. It is as though this negative energy is rarely neutralized, and more of it keeps piling up within the body. FMS is, in my view, the natural process of the nervous system gone awry.

For me, rain equals pain. I can tell today that the barometric pressure has changed. I am beginning to ache badly. When I check the forecast and see that there is 75 percent relative humidity, I know it will be a bad day. My body knows it! I feel so sick. I dread the change of seasons. I cannot tolerate intense heat, frigid cold, or humidity.

The similarities between CFS and FMS, and tangentially MCS (also known as EI, environmental illness) cannot be pushed aside. In my view, people with CFS and FMS eventually develop environmental sensitivities, and, in fact, the conditions may be precipitated by chemical or other environmental exposures. While there is little written about the commonalities between these three syndromes (except in Wallace and Wallace[1]) and Gulf War syndrome, nonetheless I believe that eventually they will be linked together in some fashion, possibly even under toxic chemical exposures as a precipitating factor for the HSP. However, it is important for me to point out here that while those with FMS also have CFS, neither of these conditions *always* have EI/MCS. Furthermore, EI/MCS can be present in a person without he or she having FMS or CFS. In my view the extreme case is the person with FMS who also has CFS (which is a given) and EI/ MCS. Perhaps it could be said that FMS and CFS are siblings while MCS is a first or even a distant cousin.

It will be important to follow the effects of the war in Iraq to assess whether or not more of these syndromes are presented. Is there any worse scenario for the person who is highly sensitive than going to, or living within, the horrors of war? Killing is not good for the nervous system (said with tongue in cheek) or, obviously and sadly, for the victims who themselves are threatened by the possibility of being killed. Their tales have yet to be systematically documented. It is little wonder that stress combined with the toxins that are emitted during combat would traumatize the nervous system of military personnel and those victims being invaded. However, is it possible that many military personnel and other victims of war develop highly sensitive personalities as a result of the chaos and pain they encounter? This is another chicken and egg dilemma for the reader to ponder. Perhaps the psychic pain and chemicals combine to produce a highly sensitive person, rather than having had the trait prior to their current situation. Another possibility is that in war there are so many toxins within the physical environment that the nature of the person plays an insignificant role in the current debate over Gulf War Syndrome. The reader will be struck throughout this book with the fact that I have more questions than answers to these perplexing issues. It is highly likely that veterans of other wars have experienced not only posttraumatic stress syndrome (PTSS) but also fibromyalgia, although not identified as such. It could be that PTSS is also a cousin to fibromyalgia. These relationships are difficult to untangle.

My view is that fibromyalgia, Gulf War syndrome, posttraumatic stress syndrome, environmental illness, and chronic fatigue syndrome should be explored via the over-aroused nervous system, which has in these cases been frequently bombarded by stimuli to the extent that psycho-social and/or environmental factors over-stimulate the autonomic nervous system. Furthermore, I believe (based upon Aron's theory of the HSP and Easterbrooks's theory of the USP) that some persons, particularly women, are born with or develop highly sensitive nervous systems that allow the person to be "aware of subtleties in the environment" (Aron's words). It is almost as if a person is born without a strong emotional immune system, which manifests itself in physical and psychological suffering, especially as the years progress. Still, while both FMS and CFS share major common symptoms, they mysteriously have some different aspects, particularly in terms of chronicity. I can provide no conclusive evidence that there is a relationship between people with fibromyalgia or chronic fatigue and heightened sensitivity to the feelings of others, and, of course, there is no absolute assurance. But I have informally asked many women about this theory, and all have agreed with it without hesitation. It does demand reflection and a different way of observing the world of those with CFS and FMS. It is a theory that could be substantiated or refuted by future research. However, my intent is to focus more specifically on FMS.

Teitelbaum[21] writes that in his practice among his patients with chronic fatigue and fibromyalgia there is a heightened sensitivity to the needs of others, which further substantiates my theory. However, I do not want to paint an entirely negative picture of this personality type. Teitelbaum and Aron both point out that there are positive aspects to being highly sensitive (such as high intelligence and inquisitiveness), and I will focus on positive characteristics in a later chapter.

A visit to the Nova Scotia Environmental Centre and discussion with Dr. Fox has reinforced my theory of the highly sensitive person. In fact, he himself has already postulated about this hypersensitivity among those clients in the centre and has presented a paper about the highly sensitive person at an international symposium. If it is true that some of us can be born with or develop highly sensitive nervous systems, it seems likely that as we continue to be bombarded with either biological or psycho-social stimuli, a breaking point occurs. This reinforces my view of the body/mind connection. I wish FMS was taken away from the arthritis specialists and given to the neurologists, to the counsellors who deal with emotional trauma, and to some complementary practitioners like massage therapists, chiropractors, and others who do body work. What we FMS sufferers need is information about how to maintain an optimal level of stimulation of the nervous system, not drugs for the symptoms. When Dr. Fox suggested Aron's book, it was as though the world of FMS suddenly became clear to me. Yes, many women are sensitive to the needs of others, but not to the extent of the HSP/USP. To even assume that all women are ultra-sensitive is an essentialist view defining all women with a single core of being. In fact, it is this ultra-sensitivity of the continuously aroused sympathetic nervous system (that part of the nervous system that brings about an acceleration of the autonomic nervous system) that I am thinking of as a predisposing factor (which children and men can also develop). Why is it though that no one has speculated about the links between fibromyalgia and exaggerated sensitivities, the nature of most women's lives, and the lives of others in crisis situations? I ask myself this question frequently.

Before I continue with the development of the theory about the over-aroused nervous system, let me now present a brief summary of relevant neuroanatomy in order to augment my thesis regarding a neuro-psychological cause. This section will be followed by specifics of pain, fatigue, and sleep disturbances, because these must be presented in more detail in order to provide a complete picture of fibromyalgia.

The nervous system

The nervous system is divided into the *central nervous system* and the *peripheral nervous system*. The central nervous system is divided into two parts: the brain and the spinal cord. The peripheral nervous system is also divided into two major parts: the somatic nervous system and the autonomic nervous system. This curt summary points out the structure of the nervous system, which, while divided into several connected systems, nonetheless functions as a whole. However, it is the autonomic nervous system, the portion of the peripheral nervous system that controls and regulates the automatic processes and functions of the body that is the focus of this analysis.

The brain contains billions of nerve cells called neurons, which make synapses with other neurons. In the case of the autonomic nervous system, neurotransmitters either cause us to "fight or take flight" (the sympathetic nervous system) and "rest and digest" (parasympathetic nervous system). The actual wiring of the brain and how it works at the highest level is not known; however, it is my contention that the autonomic nervous system of the highly sensitive person, who is on perpetual alert regarding emotional states and perceived needs of others, is herself in a constant state of long-term imbalance, which leads to exhaustion and depression, resulting in such conditions as fibromyalgia, chronic fatigue, and often subsequent multiple chemical sensitivities. It is as though this continuously antagonistic yet regulatory autonomic system, which is supposed to keep the body in balance, is in a constant state of upheaval, whereby the automatic processes are thrown into perpetual hyper-arousal.

Although this is but a cursory overview of the functions of the nervous system, it nevertheless provides the reader with some degree of understanding regarding the theory I postulate regarding the relationship between the highly sensitive person and the autonomic nervous system. What then can result from this imbalance? There are three areas that I believe are crucial to an understanding of the complex issues surrounding fibromyalgia:

- Postulated causes, which I have just discussed

- Symptoms and management of symptoms, which I will also briefly discuss in the next section and explore in more detail in subsequent chapters

- What can be done with an over-aroused nervous system when women are hesitant to put their own needs first, which will be the basis of the last chapter

While there are many symptoms of fibromyalgia, I consider pain, fatigue, and sleep disturbances to cause the most distress—although it could be argued that depression and chemical sensitivities should be listed among them. In this section, I do not discuss depression or MCS. Not all FMS sufferers are plagued with depression, but all have pain, fatigue, and sleep disturbances. Furthermore, not all have MCS, and it must be pointed out that not all persons with MCS have fibromyalgia.

Pain and FMS

Pain, whether acute or chronic, is not well understood. It is highly subjective; one may live with chronic pain for many years and continue to function adequately in daily activities, while another may be completely immobilized by it. For some, there is little relief; for others, there may be some degree of relief from an over-the-counter pain medication. Yet for others, only heavy narcotics can allow them to continue with their normal activities. Some of the literature suggests that anxiety is a precursor to pain.[22] I do not believe, however, that anxiety must always precede fibromyalgia pain. There could be multiple factors which affect the nervous system and subsequently cause pain; for example, happy excitement could cause the arousal of an over-stimulated nervous system. Still, like FMS itself, pain is indeed a complicated phenomenon.

It's late, and my back is so tired. The pain is shooting down to my hands. I must get up and move about and stretch. The thrill of believing I now understand FMS and its relationship to the sensitive nervous system keeps me writing far too long at the keyboard. I must set shorter limits for myself. But the excitement keeps me going, and I seem to feed on the stimulation. Like Dr. Teitelbaum suggests, we experience an adrenalin high. I need to give care to my own mind and body connection, or I will continue to have intense attacks.

General features of FMS pain

Generally, the most troublesome symptom for people with FMS is widespread pain, usually described as "sore all over." This complaint most often results in a referral to a rheumatologist. Usually, pain and stiffness, present upon awakening, gradually improve into the early afternoon. Simms, reporting on the laboratory studies of the muscles of people with FMS, describes them as "moth eaten" and "ragged-red" muscle fibers.[23] The latter description evokes images I personally can relate to, particularly as I often imagine the pain as constant fire in my muscles, a demon that never leaves me. Other times, there are sharp shock-like pains that cause me to gasp out loud, which is different from the fire imagery.

Karen Moore Schaefer[24] cites the kinds of pain described by the women in her study of FMS. They used words such as bad, nagging, unremitting, agony, terrible, annoying, burning, and extreme. Among women with FMS, there are many varied interpretations of pain, often differing by race, ethnicity, age, class, physical or mental abilities, and other variables. I speculate that because many women have been subjected to so much emotional as well as physical pain in their lives, they often find it difficult to describe. Furthermore, women often bury or ignore their pain, or come to believe it is natural. I believe that there are many more women out there who have FMS but have stoically hidden their condition as they attend to the affective needs of others and fear that they will not meet those needs.

Treatment for pain

Because the people with FMS are responsible for self reporting their own pain, which is subjective and interpreted differently by those who experience it, the idea of quantifying pain for regulation is impossible. Both nurses and doctors are subject to the scientific-medical discourse of pain and its management, which includes numerical and adjectival rating scales and face scales.[25] Yet people respond differently to pain and therefore cannot describe its manifestations to anyone else completely adequately. This causes disparity between the medical view and the personal experience, especially when some people hide or bury the intensity of their pain. Medical practitioners can be prone to disputing the very existence of the pain, while patients are either trying to prove they are suffering or dismissing it as some shortcoming of their own. Women, generally looking out for the needs of others, are less likely to report pain if they believe that it will disadvantage others. In fact, the women in this study relayed stories about concealing their pain from loved ones or colleagues.

I rarely told anyone I worked with that I have FMS . Consequently, I did not have any excuse for not overworking, often in a stressful atmosphere. Why was I ashamed of it? I have found the words of Dr. Teitelbaum to be helpful: "No blame, no fault, no guilt, no judgement, make no comparisons." I must be a friend to myself.

The patterns of FMS vary from person to person, and many suffer for years without relief. Others become experts of their own bodies and begin to understand what causes flare-ups. However, it must be recognized that there is chronic as well as acute pain. Some of us become so adjusted to chronic pain that it becomes secondary to our lives. An acute flare-up is something new to deal with, particularly as the nature of an acute attack can vary. Sometimes the pain is a dull ache, while other times it is excruciating. Because of this variability, it is necessary to understand the differences and how to treat the pain. Chaitow[4] describes various pain pattern treatments like pain-killing injections, acupressure, acupuncture, electrotherapy, and other such practices that I will describe in more detail in chapter 6. One of the newer treatments that proclaims to be effective for FMS is Vitalaxin 20, which contains porcine relaxin, a polypeptide insulin-like hormone. Various Web pages with more information about Vitalaxin can be found on the Internet. I personally have not taken it, and I do not know anyone who has. This, however, is but one of many pain-control drugs like, for example, Neurontin (Gabapentin), which are said to control neuropathic pain and may help with fibromyalgia. Some take such substances as OxyContin and morphine. These are only a few in a myriad of medications that may help some and may be useless for others. How do sufferers know what to try? Pain control is often in the hands of the physician, who can prescribe the medications. But how do we make sense of the confusion regarding the cause of the pain?

Those electric shocks that go through me are the worst. I can barely keep from yelping aloud. But today it is a dull ache everywhere, feeling like the flu. Sometimes it is mental anguish that I feel because I think this will never leave me completely. Is there anything that will give relief? So far nothing has really had any long-term effects. So many things cause these acute attacks.

Looking to soothe the effects of pain is a necessary but short-sighted solution. Instead of spending so much time trying to find something that will alleviate the discomfort, why not expend the energy to explore what is causing it to occur in the first place? Clearly, more appropriate research into the causes of chronic and acute pain in fibromyalgia patients is required if we are to actually cure it. And as Teitelbaum has pointed out, there is a definite mind/body connection. The complexity of the issues is mind boggling.

Fatigue and FMS

Fatigue, like pain, is a symptom not a disease, and the description of it is often contextually bound by such variables as class, gender, race, ethnicity, lifestyle (particularly occupation), and age. Also, like pain, it is an elusive concept that can only be described qualitatively and subjectively. Hart and Grace[26] point out that exploring fatigue is problematic since it is so ill-defined. It can arise from many conditions and is said to be one of the most common symptoms related by patients to medical professionals. With regard to women, fatigue becomes extremely difficult to explore because it is often associated with other kinds of distress such as the double jeopardy of home and work, lack of sleep, depression, and other stressors, especially if the woman is a highly sensitive person. This fatigue is not just tiredness in the usual sense of the word; it is extremely debilitating and can be triggered by many kinds of stimulation of the nervous system. It is usually the first symptom of CFS.

I remember my first experience of fatigue. I was walking around the water-front with my three young sons and thought I was about to collapse. The fatigue so overwhelmed me that I had to lie on a bench, much to the children's dismay. Little did I know that it would probably last a lifetime, although not appearing often or to such a dramatic extent.

It is with the description of fatigue that the differences between chronic fatigue and fibromyalgia begin to blur. I believe that if the two were to be separated then there may be an artificial distinction. Yet I have seen CFS symptoms disappear forever, whereas FMS appears to last a lifetime. CFS is defined primarily as an illness [sic] whose etiology is not definitely known, that primarily affects women, and has been thought by many to be caused by a virus.[27] It has bred the idea that since women are more affected there must therefore be a psychiatric explanation; that is, it is the result of the woman's inadequacies. Hence, the personality theory evolved, thereby disputing the idea of a viral causation. There is an ongoing search for a cause of CFS. The failure to find a specific viral etiology for CFS supported by all researchers resulted in the psychologization of the condition. Tarred with this same brush are environmental illness, (often called multiple chemical sensitivities), and fibromyalgia. Although not as widely discussed, with this trio is the reflex sympathetic dystrophy/complex regional pain syndrome (RSD/CRPS), a condition that appears to be an exaggerated form of FMS and CFS and also affects predominantly women. I will not discuss the latter in greater detail, but there are Web sites available for those who want to know more about it.

As long ago as 1991, Bell[28] wrote that doctors often inappropriately treated those suffering from chronic fatigue with mood-altering drugs or advocated more exercise than the patients were able to handle while at the same time under-prescribing medications for pain relief. Some actually believe that because there were more women competing with men in the job market that women were unable to handle the pressure. It can be argued that, in fact, women have had to carry on with their home and job responsibilities, often as single parents also caring for aged parents or other family members. With little help in the home, they therefore become chronically tired and have nervous systems that are constantly in a state of over-arousal. Rather than psychologizing women, it is more reasonable to place the responsibility on societal expectations of women. The process of developing FMS and CFS is contextual and relational in my view. While the end result may be that women need counselling, physical assistance with responsibilities to overcome these pressures, and help in calming their over-aroused nervous systems, it is unreasonable to place the blame on those who suffer. Few women can meet the demands of our stressful society when the expectations far exceed that which are healthy. The plight of women who are expected to take care of others before their own needs are met is showing up in the growing (and alarming) numbers of women who are suffering from FMS and CFS. The fatigue of these women is more than just being tired; it is an exhaustion resulting from over caring for others, resulting in an overly alert sympathetic nervous system.

Being tired differs from chronic fatigue, and unless someone has experienced both, the differences cannot be clearly explained. The language does not exist. Words are often inadequate. Unlike for pain, there is little Western medical treatment for fatigue. Homeopathic solutions and complementary therapies, including vitamin and mineral supplements, are usually final resorts when all else has failed. Sometimes, happily, there will be a dramatic change, but there is growing evidence that this is a coincidental placebo effect. Generally though, in the view that I am postulating, I believe that the actual hands-on treatments such as massage, chiropractic manipulation, and acupuncture will not be effective in the long term unless the person develops an awareness of the body/mind connection and the extent to which the stimulation of the nervous system leads to physiological over-arousal. The end result is pain and fatigue.

Fatigue criteria

While the most significant information about fatigue is found in the writings about CFS, I believe that FMS sufferers experience the same kind of fatigue. I therefore present here the criteria that is noted in the Skelly and Helm text.[29] They write that the fatigue must

- Be of at least six months duration;

- Not be lifelong (i.e. the person must remember feeling "normal");

- Result in a substantial reduction of occupational, educational, social, or personal activities as compared to the person's activities before the onset of illness;

- Not be the result of ongoing exertion or be relieved by rest.

Furthermore, as pointed out by Goldberg[30] chronic fatigue is accompanied by pain, headaches, and poor concentration. It is "an umbrella term for a multiple symptom disorder." Therefore, fatigue, like pain, cannot be viewed in isolation of other symptoms, and one cannot manage the symptoms without viewing the gestalt.

Sleep Disturbances

In her book *The Fibromyalgia Advocate*, Starlanyl[11] writes:

> People with FMS often have the alpha-delta sleep anomaly. During delta sleep, bodies heal, and many neurotransmitters are restored to health. As soon as you reach deep delta-level sleep, alpha waves, which characterize the awake state, intrude and either jolt you to awakening or to a lighter stage of sleep. You wake up feeling as if you've been run over by a truck. When you are deprived of sleep, the deep delta-level healing processes are cut short before they can do their work.

Sleep ties in with my ever-growing view of the over-stimulated nervous system, which cannot settle. This again leads to my belief that one cannot find a medical model answer to these complex, medically constructed symptoms. In my view, it is the parasympathetic nervous system's inability to tone down the body.

Starlanyl also writes about restless leg syndrome, which often occurs with FMS usually just before or during sleep and is one of the automatic nervous system peculiarities. Often, sleep is disrupted by these leg sensations. This unpleasant syndrome results in being unable to keep legs quieted as they ache due to a sensation of heaviness and/or twitching that is often difficult to describe to others. Nocturnal cramps (myoclonus) are also often part of the process of trying to fall asleep, which I again attribute to over-stimulation of the nervous system in a highly sensitive person.

It's starting again; I need a hot bath. It feels like my legs cannot be still. I don't have the words to describe this squirming or twitching that seems so deep in my legs. I'm reading the words of Elaine Scarry where she talks about the "unsharability" of the language of pain. One of my massage therapists says it is the central nervous system discharging through the sympathetic nervous system. That explanation feels right to me, but if someone has not experienced it, I can-

not describe what it feels like! It's not exactly pain but extreme discomfort that interferes with my sleep.

The twilight sleep that many FMS patients complain of is debilitating. The nerve impulses do not seem to stop, even when the patient is asleep, and the person is left fatigued in the morning. I liken this to the half-awake/half-asleep sensation that often occurs during a daytime catnap.

Simms[31] writes that both amitriptyline and cyclobenzaprine are antidepressant drugs that also appear to be effective for sleep disturbances. Taken in low doses, they appear to help with sleep disorders. While there are natural substances that can be taken in place of these chemicals, I will discuss them in a subsequent chapter.

Conclusion

There are many other symptoms that are integral to FMS—depression, intestinal upsets, itchy skin, and headaches among others—but I have chosen here to focus primarily on the three main ones. It is important to recognize that none of them can be treated in isolation of the other. All must be regarded as interrelated. Sleep, pain, fatigue, and other debilitating characteristics of FMS will appear in subsequent chapters as I let the voices of the women relate how they manage their everyday lives.

While this chapter does not include each and every article and book that has been written on the symptoms of fibromyalgia (or indeed the topic of fibromyalgia itself), I have chosen instead to focus on those professionals who have written the most about the condition. The Internet alone cites hundreds of articles and books, a list too extensive to include in a book of this nature. Few books, however, include the voices of the women themselves who are experts of their own experiences with FMS. I will turn now to the women and describe some of their characteristics so that the reader can begin to know a little about their lived experiences.

2

Meet the Women

In this chapter, I will introduce the twenty women who shared their stories for this book. I have given them fictitious names to protect their identities. There are women from British Columbia, Ontario, and Nova Scotia, Canada. Fourteen women are white, and six are black. The women were generally chosen through a "snowball" technique; that is, one woman would tell me about another woman she knew who also had fibromyalgia. In some instances, friends or relatives would give me someone's name. In three cases, I already knew the person as a friend or colleague. Each woman I did not know was initially contacted by a familiar person who knew me in order to seek her willingness to participate in an extensive face-to-face interview with me. I did not directly contact an unknown woman until I had been given permission to do so by the middle person. After the taped interviews were transcribed, I gave each woman a copy of the transcription. In the case of e-mail, which I used with some of the participants for additional information, I preserved the data with the other transcripts. I also sent the participants rough copies of several chapters and asked for them to give me some feedback regarding how they were depicted. In addition, I asked them to comment on my theory regarding why women were more prone to fibromyalgia. Those who responded (all but three of the women) told me they agreed completely with my theory about the highly sensitive person and an overstimulated nervous system.

At the university where I was employed, I presented a research proposal about this research to the ethics committee and received permission to proceed. The women signed a consent form indicating their willingness to take part in this qualitative study. Because I was using myself as one of the participants, I was interviewed by one of the other women. This is a very subjective piece of work, as only those who have lived through the day-to-day drama of fibromyalgia are qualified to speak of living the experience.

As a white woman, I acknowledge that I am in a position of privilege by virtue of my white skin and academic credentials, and this could have created bias in interviewing. Nonetheless, the stories that all the women shared with me are so similar that it seemed reasonable to me that, aside from racism (which I acknowledge is a huge factor to consider), we all experienced at least the same physical and emotional challenges. I also recognize that the lives of black women are infinitely more difficult in a racist society, and I am in danger of minimizing this suffering by lumping black and white women together as if we all experience FMS in the same way. I have attempted to be as sensitive to this issue as possible. I found that economic insecurities were extremely important to many of the women; my sample includes a cross-section of people from diverse class backgrounds. As I share a profile of each woman, understand that we all have had to redesign our lives in many ways. While all of the women gave informed consent to be interviewed, I nonetheless refrain from giving too much detail regarding their backgrounds. I will, however, detail my own life as it ties in to my theory of FMS and HSP. I believe that all of us who suffer from psychic and/or physical pain long to tell our stories, as it is in the telling that there is some degree of comfort and release.

Jean

At the time of the original interview, Jean was fifty-four years old. She is a retired school teacher who is white and of mainly Scottish background. She has been told that multiple sclerosis, which she has had since she was twenty-nine, is more common among people whose ancestors come from Scotland. She retired at age fifty because of multiple sclerosis. At around the age of forty-one, she was told by her neurologist that she had fibromyalgia. Because of the similarities of the two conditions, she is never quite sure if the symptoms she experiences are MS or FMS, but her physician told her that much of the pain and discomfort she experienced was, in fact, caused by FMS.

Jean lives in a small town with her spouse, also a retired school teacher, and has two married sons and several grandchildren. She defines her mother as a highly sensitive person who sacrifices herself for others, and she believes she has acquired that same characteristic. She has contact with the formal health-care system through Western-trained medical physicians; she also works with complementary therapists. She describes herself as extremely sensitive to people's needs and emotions, and she is easily emotionally hurt by others, readily becomes anxious, and cannot tolerate confrontation or conflict. She anticipates what others are thinking and "feels their energy." Formerly, she had high levels of energy, but now she does not have the same mobility, is mostly wheelchair bound, and has found that her lifestyle has changed dramatically as a result. She worked hard and was conscientious about her work with the children she taught. Each project she completed was followed by a bigger and more labour-intensive one. Jean described herself as somewhat of a perfectionist but noted that she attended to the needs of others before her own, particularly those of the children she taught. While she could move about somewhat with two canes, she uses either a scooter or wheelchair outside the home. She needs a great deal of contact with the outside world and often pushes herself to go out. This is often difficult as she is highly sensitive to the impact she might be having on others, particularly as they see her in a wheelchair, and she is always highly tuned to what others may be thinking. She goes to great lengths not to offend others.

Jean is socially active and very religious. She finds prayer to be the most helpful to her during stressful times. She takes numerous vitamins and supplements, has visited a chiropractor, has occasional massages, has had 'cleansing' on the advice of a herbalist, and has had electrotherapy, which she found somewhat temporarily helpful for pain. Her most troublesome symptoms are sleeping disorders, pain, fatigue, and depression, which also affect her walking. She takes medication for depression, occasionally Elavil for sleep, and other MS medications.

Amy

Amy is a forty-six-year-old white woman who lives with her spouse in a large city and is a professor in an administrative position with a high degree of status. She has not had any children. Amy says she felt "crummy" about 60 percent of the time while working in a high-stress job. Upon looking back, she believes she began having symptoms of FMS in 1992, but she was officially diagnosed in 1995. She thinks that FMS developed after a particularly bad bout of a virus. She "felt terrible, and, of course, I had been working as hard as I could while I was feeling terrible."

Amy describes herself as once having had enormous amounts of energy; she would push herself to extremes at whatever she attempted. She describes having most of the common symptoms of FMS, but she says that fatigue (which she described as "crushing") is the worst, as it depletes her energy. She was "hard driving," even more so on herself than on others. When she finds herself having a bad day, she relies on "strong mental discipline" and tells herself, "You're going to push through this." She is convinced that high stress results in a neurochemical imbalance, which, she believes, is a probable cause of FMS.

"I take vitamins religiously," she tells me. She also takes St. John's wort and often has massages. She practices imaging to calm her racing mind, which seems to be in constant motion. She pushes herself through crippling bouts of lack of mobility to extreme limits in order to fulfill obligations, despite difficulty concentrating, a major symptom of depression. She is highly sensitive to the needs of others in spite of her physical limitations. She is a caretaker in her professional life, and she is in tune with the energy in a room. She dislikes conflict and is very sensitive to it in her environment. Yet in spite of intense bouts of fibromyalgia, she carries on daily with her high-powered job and does not give in to the chronic pain, even when she is using canes to move about. She says she is extremely stoic and does not discuss her condition openly with many people. Raised in poverty, she is proud of her accomplishments and status.

Leanne

Leanne, a black woman, is one of the youngest of our group. At age thirty-seven at the time of the first interview, she was working full time as a counsellor for black students. Her job required intense compassion for students, combating racism, and struggling to improve the plight of black students in a racist society. Leanne's work required her to take on racist policies, subtle or overt within the workplace. Because of her sensitive nature, she oftentimes found herself embroiled in situations that were unhealthy for her emotionally.

Her office had been remade into a scent-free environment, and, by her own admission, it was oftentimes difficult to find physical places where her symptoms were not intensified. She believes that she had environmental illness long before she was diagnosed and knows that it is related to fibromyalgia. She believes she had FMS even as a child living in a predominantly white community with few black people. She has many health problems, which were misdiagnosed in the past. In particular, she has a serious sleeping disorder, depression, fatigue, and pain.

Although she does not specifically identify herself as psychologically sensitive, she says she is always able to pick up on people's moods and differentiate between types of people whom she calls "nice" or "genuine" or "nasty." She too is greatly in tune with the energy in a room. She also says she often has deja vu. Leanne believes that we are predisposed to FMS, or perhaps it is hereditary.

Leanne had a job that was high stress and high profile. She lives in a city with her spouse and has not had any children. She often found it difficult to take what she called "medical holidays," but immediately after our first interview, she ended up on long-term disability. She says that her best results for symptom relief come from complementary medicines. While she would like to work part time, she does not believe she could afford to keep up with her medications if she did so and is uncertain about her professional future. She is currently very ill, unable to work, and at times housebound. This is very unsettling for a once high-energy person. Complicating her alienation while housebound are bouts of acute depression and a myriad of other disabling symptoms.

Anna

At forty-eight, Anna found that she could no longer work full time as a dental assistant. Her symptoms began in the winter of 1994 following a car accident, but she was only officially diagnosed in 1999. She is now working part time as a receptionist. Anna is a white woman who lives with her spouse and two teenagers in a city. She keeps herself busy at home doing craftwork because she enjoys it and because it helps to keep her fingers mobile as she experiences hand and joint pain.

Anna describes herself as an outgoing person who loves helping people. She said she used to be a "bubbly type person" who has "gone quieter" as a result of FMS. She used to be "restless" but has found that her personality changed because of frequent exhaustion. She was once a hard-driving working person who now feels "burnt out." She used to entertain regularly but rarely does so now. Of the complementary therapies, she has tried electromagnetic therapy by wearing small discs on her body, and she takes vitamins and has had massages. But she is not convinced any of these modalities are effective in the long term. She is acutely aware of the needs of other people, and that is why she chose a profession whereby she could help others. She has become very sensitive to complaining about her distress with FMS. She does not like to discuss her symptoms with her immediate family because she believes it upsets them, and she is unwilling to bore them with talk of the pain she is experiencing. Upsetting and sensing discomfort in others with her complaints was stressful for her.

Vera

Vera is a fifty-six-year-old white woman who lives with her spouse in a city. She does not have any children or any close family members. She has recently retired from her job as manager in an office. During the economic climate of cutbacks, she worked under a great deal of stress. After twenty-five years in the same job, she felt she was badly treated by a new director, and the stress of this continued for some time. She was referred by this new boss to a psychologist, and she felt it was "degrading" because everyone knew about her situation. Always feeling that she was in tune with what other people were thinking about her, she became embarrassed about her job situation and very sensitive about the atmosphere in her work-place. She believes that several circumstances precipitated her FMS: intense care-giving for a mother who was ill and for whom she was totally responsible, marrying at a late age (even though it was a happy occasion, it was difficult to live with someone else later in life), the work environment, a car accident and the resultant whiplash, and a hysterectomy.

Vera takes antioxidant vitamins, visits a naturopath, has physiotherapy and acupuncture treatments, takes various herbs, and is on an antidepressant. She has many chemical sensitivities, and humid weather is very difficult for her. She believes that, after moving to an air-tight building at work, she began to suffer from symptoms more often.

She describes herself as someone whose feelings are easily hurt and says she is "not a fighter." Vera does not like arguments or conflict. In short, she has a sensitive nature and says that she "wounds easy." Although her home is her castle, she is in it more than she wants to be, but weather changes were especially difficult for her, and she is often housebound.

Becky

Becky, a forty-three-year-old white woman, was married at the time of the interview but subsequently divorced from her spouse. She has two teenagers who then lived with her alone in a city. She is a nurse who is now back at work after taking sick leave. She believes that she developed FMS after a hysterectomy several years ago.

During her childhood, her mother would tell her she was like a "hot-house plant" because she always needed tender care and was never able to push herself to extreme limits. She has always been labelled as "being too sensitive, hypersensitive." She has always tried "to meet the expectations at home, running the house and being there for the children and doing my work and being something for everybody." She describes her father as "sensitive to woes" and "a very tender-heart type of man" who died of a massive heart attack at age sixty. His death was traumatic for her as she lost the one person who could relate to her emotional sensitivities and vulnerability.

Becky believes that there is a mind/body connection with FMS. She thinks that people with FMS are "thinkers, feelers, sometimes of a more quiet personality ... they're more in tune with themselves." She believes that FMS burns out the body quickly. She is agitated by too much stimuli and hates too much pressure. She has environmental sensitivities now that she did not have before. She says that "everything in my body is hypersensitive now."

While Becky does not engage in any kind of complementary therapy with professionals, she does hand exercises and massages her own neck and hands. In addition, she uses magnetic therapy and has had good success with pain control. She sleeps under a far-infrared quilt on a magnetic mattress and pillow. She also uses magnetic insoles, necklaces, bracelets, and earrings, all of which help her tremendously. She finds peace through meditation and reading the Bible, and she tries to avoid too much stimulation, although this is very difficult sometimes in her workplace.

Sally

Sally, a forty-four-year-old white woman, lives in a city and has a part-time nursing job. She lives with her spouse and does not have children. Following the stress of her father's death, a viral infection, poor working conditions, and a car accident, she was diagnosed with FMS.

"I'm a worrier ... I worry for everybody, not just myself. And a lot of times, I don't worry about myself the way I should. I'm too busy worrying about other people. I don't like to do things wrong." Sally feels she is *overly* sensitive to not doing the right thing for others. Not only does she describe herself as highly sensitive, but she believes she is psychic. By this she means she gets feelings that she cannot describe and seems to know when things aren't right. She says that as a child "even though I was asleep, I was always aware of what was going on around me. I suppose I do the same now." More succinctly, she was always in a state of emotional hyperarousal. Her feelings are easily hurt, and she does not like noise or confusion. She says she is definitely a sensitive person who always wants to push herself further for others. She recognizes that she reacts strongly to stimuli, whether in response to the emotions of others or within her own body in the form of chemical and food sensitivities, especially dairy products. She also suffers from asthma.

While she believes there are remissions for FMS, she thinks that certain personality types are prone to it. She says she takes care of the needs of others before herself. For her own benefit, she practices imagery and takes various vitamins. She suffers from pain, fatigue, and sleep disturbances.

Louise

Louise is a white woman who lives in a city with her spouse. She has one married daughter and grandchildren. She was fifty-five years old at the time of the first interview. She was diagnosed with FMS when she was about forty-nine after she was told she had polymyalgia. She was on sick leave at the time of the interview, after working in several careers, the last one in an office. She described that her "personality is to push, push, push, push." If the work is to be done in three hours, she wants to do it in two. She says that she cannot do the things she used to do, and excitement causes her to feel anxious. If something is not done immediately, she worries about it; she is an "extremist." She says that she worries about the smallest task and wants it to be over with so she can get on with the next one, a major issue for those who suffer from generalized anxiety.

Louise takes various supplements and has had physiotherapy as well as the occasional massage. She swims regularly in spite of the pain and has occasionally used a cane in the past. She misses riding her bike around the city and working outside the home. Recently, however, she has returned to part-time office work.

She does not see her grandchildren regularly because the stimulation is difficult for her and increases her pain, fatigue, and sleep disturbances. She describes herself as burnt out.

Germaine

Germaine lives in a big city, owns a beauty salon, and supervises a large staff. At age fifty-six, she lives with her spouse and does not have children. She says her attack came on suddenly several years ago, totally incapacitating her body. "And I am a very, very active person—energy very, very high." She now has three people doing the job she used to do alone. Since the onset of FMS, she is highly sensitive to noise and prefers quieter surroundings. She said that for thirty-six years she worked hard physically and mentally for sixteen hours a day and seven days a week; "I really drove myself." Germaine tells me that she hasn't seen too many people who had the stamina she once had.

Originally from Germany, Germaine, a white woman, returns to Europe often, where she goes to a spa and has lymphatic massage, which helps her tremendously. Germaine suffers from restless legs and is unable to sleep well. As a result, she is usually very fatigued and has a great deal of pain. She does, however, take a special kind of 'Noni' juice from Tahiti that she says helps her energy level.

When asked if she thinks there is a specific FMS personality type, she says she thinks there are those "who have a very high energy level, are in an environment where there is lots of noise and action." She believes that too much stimuli is responsible for FMS. In addition, as I watched her in her workplace, I perceived that she feels tremendous responsibility for her staff and clients, who confide in her as a mother figure. I was able to see how adroitly she anticipates the slightest needs of those around her.

Diane

Diane, a fifty-four-year-old white woman, lives with her spouse in a small town and has multiple sclerosis. She had MS symptoms at age twenty-three and, at forty-eight, developed FMS. Her children are grown and have left home. She describes herself as having been a "supermom." Following a hysterectomy, she became sensitive to mould and perfume and had to leave her job in a textile factory. FMS developed a few days after the surgery.

At one time, she would have described herself as pushing too hard, unable to pace herself. Now she has to slow down and not push because the MS and FMS will not allow it. Diane has been to a naturopath, does vitamin therapy, and has learned therapeutic touch. She uses other complementary approaches to help herself. She has changed her eating habits, and she exercises when she is able. She was close to her elderly mother, who recently died, which has been a very stressful experience. On some days, her MS is invisible, and she is able to carry out her activities easily. But weather changes and especially environmental sensitivities to perfume and other chemicals affect her dramatically.

She suffers from incapacitating pain, fatigue, and multiple chemical sensitivities. Ongoing contact with her reveals that she continues to feel less well over time.

Candace

Candace, a white, forty-seven-year-old woman, is a flight attendant who lives in a small village with her spouse. She has never had children. She was diagnosed with FMS several years ago after a vicious viral infection that left her paralyzed from the neck down for a few hours. She describes FMS as stress related and "doing too much." She says that although she used to have a great deal of energy, she doesn't anymore. Her days are spent anticipating the needs of others as her job demands.

When she was a small girl, if there was going to be an event in the school, she would get sick; that is, she was very sensitive to unusual circumstances in the form of too much stimuli. "I'll go till I can't go anymore," she says as she speaks of pushing herself beyond her limits. She had been having anxiety attacks and chest pain due to stress, and she is very subject to colds and flu, possibly caused by the air quality in a plane, which exacerbate her symptoms of FMS.

Candace takes many vitamins and other supplements and visits a naturopath. In addition, she has massages. Like many of the women, she takes Echinacea regularly to help build up her immune system. Her acute attacks of fibromyalgia are becoming more and more debilitating.

Michelle

Michelle is a thirty-five-year-old black woman who lives with her two teenage children in a city. She believes she began having symptoms at age eighteen after giving birth to her first child. She believes that she developed environmental illness from contaminants while working in a factory. She lost her full-time job because of downsizing, and she now works on occasion as a postal worker. Otherwise, she receives social assistance.

Prior to FMS and the development of her many chemical sensitivities, Michelle "was always on the go." She was fanatical about house cleaning, but now she can barely keep up. She says that she usually did not take a great deal of time to take care of herself. Now, she finds that she has changed tremendously. She is not able to go out frequently, and her desire for a social life has diminished. She describes herself as a super-organized perfectionist who used to scrub the floors everyday. Now, she has to force herself to go out and feels guilty if the house is not extremely tidy. In short, she suffered from anxiety that precipitated pain, insomnia, and gastrointestinal problems.

Michelle tries to do a Tae-Bo exercise video, though kickboxing is difficult. She tells me that she often feels like she is on an emotional roller coaster, particularly as she and her daughter have so many environmental sensitivities. She cannot afford any complementary therapies. She is extremely concerned about the well-being of her daughters and the needs of her adoptive parents. Raised in a small, rural, white community by white parents, she became extremely sensitive to racial differences and, as a result, is a very intuitive woman.

Lesa

Lesa is a fifty-one-year-old illustrator who works at home. She is a white woman who lives alone in a city. Her FMS developed gradually about five years ago, at the time of a break-up with a partner. Even though she does aerobics and aqua-aerobics regularly, she admits it hurts her afterward. Lesa was a dancer and is keen on keeping in good physical shape.

She describes herself as a worrier who keeps things inside, as she does not like to show she is worried or upset. She cannot tolerate confrontation and says, "I am always putting myself in other people's positions." She imagines what others feel and explains, "I get myself all bound up in this, and I have, I imagine, those scenarios, and I go through them to the bitter end in my head so I know how to conduct myself." Even as a younger woman, she could not go to concerts because of the noise. She said, "I just couldn't stand noise and crowds." She is not an angry person, just easily hurt and sensitive.

After her relationship ended and she was alone in the house, she realized that another flare-up coincided with worry, especially about money. She wishes but cannot afford to eat organically, particularly as she does not qualify for unemployment insurance. She suffers a great deal of pain in her hands and feet, and worries that she will lose use of her hands and, thus, become unable to earn a living. Other than $B_{12,}$ she cannot afford any complementary therapies.

Margot

Margot is a black woman who lives with her four children in a city. She was a personal-care worker in a nursing home early in her career and then studied for one year to become a certified nursing assistant in a detox centre. However, she has not worked since 1993. She enjoyed her work but was unable to continue as FMS had become very debilitating. She was forty-two years old at the time of the first interview, with a three-year-old child and three teenagers.

"I am very sensitive to other people's feelings," she describes. A caregiver for others, she thinks of other people's needs before her own and can easily tell when there is conflict, which makes her uncomfortable. She does not easily tolerate being in environments where there is "bad energy." Because of noise, confusion, and other people's emotions, which she can usually sense, she is somewhat of a recluse.

Margot suffers from depression and says only her children keep her from committing suicide. Because of limited finances, Margot cannot afford any kind of complementary therapies. She misses working very much. Due to many chemical sensitivities, she has become quite alienated from others, in spite of being what she termed a high-energy person in the past. Her three teenage children take responsibility for running the home.

Robyn

Robyn is a fifty-one-year-old divorced white woman living in a city. She has one grown son. Following a car accident, she was forced to give up a very high-paying job as the owner of her own business. She is now so debilitated that she lives on a very reduced income with help from family members. She had lived alone until she took in a boarder. She is especially talented searching for information about fibromyalgia on the Internet and has learned a great deal about FMS.

Robyn describes herself as a Type-A personality. "I was constantly active, always on the go." She was especially active in sports and an "aggressive worker." She explains that her personality has changed dramatically; she now hates groups, is somewhat housebound, and experiences bouts of panic. She can sense the energy in a room and is sensitive to the way people are responding to one another. She also has allergies that are more serious than mere environmental sensitivities.

Robyn has had massages and physiotherapy and has researched various supplements on the Internet, but she is unable to have massages regularly or buy supplements because of her economic situation. She uses soothing essential oils, ginger, or Epsom salts in her bath. She has also studied Tai Chi and stretches every day. She would advise anyone with FMS to see a naturopath if they can afford it. Concerned about finances, she became a superintendent of the apartment complex where she was living. She is deeply reflective about fibromyalgia and explores its theories and causes as much as possible given her physical challenges.

Mandy

Mandy is a fifty-year-old black woman who has owned her own bakery and cafe and is a church organist. She has grown children and lives with her spouse in a city. She has facilitated many presentations on fibromyalgia and is well informed about it. It was from her that I first learned to recognize FMS as a psycho-neurological disorder. Mandy is asthmatic. Her own FMS symptoms developed after a severe fall left her left arm completely disabled. As a result of that accident, she has reflex sympathetic dystrophy. Because this condition appears to be an exaggerated form of FMS, she has trouble separating them. Mandy is an expert on chronic pain, belongs to a support group for chronic pain, and has traveled to Washington and Toronto to visit chronic pain centres. She does not personally believe that there is a specific kind of personality among FMS sufferers, but she has read that FMS patients have high-energy personalities.

When asked to describe herself, Mandy says that she was a high-energy person, always looking after things and people, but that she has changed because of her disabilities. She says she was a high achiever and was used to "going, going, going." She now must use a cane for walking and battles chemical sensitivities and asthma. She uses a TENS machine for pain, but she does not partake in any complementary therapies. She is searching for a biomedical explanation for FMS.

Jane

Jane was a medical laboratory technician who experienced environmental illness in the building where she worked. For nine years, she was unable to return to that building as she and many of her coworkers had become ill from "sick building syndrome." She is a forty-two-year-old black, single woman who lives alone on a long-term-disability pension. She cannot separate CFS, FMS, and MCS (or EI) symptoms from one another, as she has all three conditions.

When asked to describe herself, Jane says that she is a caregiver to everyone she cares about, is outgoing, and, in the past, always had a great deal of energy. She explains that she cares for other people's needs before her own. She will get out of a sick bed to go attend to the needs of another and has done so many times. She is a very sensitive person who removes herself from "bad energy" in a room. She has been in situations "where it's been really high energy in terms of negative energy, and I can explode ... then after I explode, it's like, you don't, you're just drained, totally drained. And then I have to go to bed." She has multiple sensitivities but does not use complementary therapies. She credits her psychiatrist for her ability to carry on from day to day in the face of great hardships. She has high regard for him and his ability to help her cope with her difficulties.

Kerry

Kerry is a forty-five-year-old black woman living in a city with a teenage son and a five-year-old son. She was a secretary in an office in a large health centre when many of the secretaries developed EI. She had been attending an environmental health centre for five years and had been off work due to illness for six years. She has complied with the therapies of the centre, has taken multiple vitamins and supplements, and has followed other kinds of therapies, such as a dry sauna. She has struggled with long-term disability (LTD) and finally won her appeal. She has many chemical sensitivities and cannot differentiate FMS from MCS. She is extremely supportive of the centre and says it has helped her tremendously. In particular, she practices an approach to healthy living called "freeze frame," a self-taught method of learning to place oneself in positive emotional states.

Describing herself as someone who pushes "as much as I can," she finds that this makes her more ill. She said that she was a very organized person until her illness. Jane is a person who keeps her feelings to herself, and she still tries "to keep a smile" even when depressed so that she does not impose her negative feelings on others. She becomes very upset if her home is not orderly and tidy. She is quick to discern moods of others, and for that reason she does not burden others with her challenges.

Maddy

Maddy is a fifty-eight-year-old white woman who lives with her spouse in a small city. She has two grown daughters. A professor, she is currently retired on long-term disability as she suffers extreme muscle cramping (tetany) of the legs as well as other body pain and fatigue, which are extremely debilitating. She was diagnosed at fifty-two, even though she had suffered from sleeplessness and depression for several years prior. She traces the FMS back to 1980 after a severe bout of mononucleosis and a bleeding ulcer.

Maddy is very reflective about FMS and attributes it "to a lifetime of surviving and high stress, demand without respite." She is a self-described highly sensitive person and understands the psychological basis for her FMS. She says, "Emotionally and socially, I have a history of being vulnerable to bullies ... abusive others, including husbands and partners and some women ... and living up to others' expectations and never feeling I really had the right to be alive." Maddy believes that there is a relationship between her sensitive nature and past psychological trauma.

EMDR (eye movement desensitization reprocessing) is a psychotherapeutic technique for dealing with past trauma. Strong pain killers, including OxyContin and morphine, and other mixes of medications are among the treatments that she has received. Currently, Codeine Contin (known as OxyContin), which is released slowly into the body and to provide relief for up to twelve hours, has been the most effective for her pain. She has traveled extensively and tried many of the treatment regimes that have been suggested to her in different countries. Always very athletic, she has been told that she has abused her body over the years. Still, she recognizes that she endured much psychological trauma in her early life, which has had a profound effect on her health. She has frequent massages, meets regularly with a certified trauma therapist, and has had joint manipulation from an osteopath. She has also taken a "biostructural" medicine called "Recovery," a disease-modifying anti-catabolic agent consisting of polyphenolic compounds.

Barbara

When I asked Amy, one of the other participants, to interview me for my book, I was sixty years old. I live in Halifax, Nova Scotia, and I have retired as a university professor. I live with my spouse, also a retired professor; our children are grown and have left home. I believe it was preordained that I would develop FMS, as I am the child of a highly sensitive mother.

Raised in Montreal, I lived in an apartment on the busiest street of that city. During my childhood, terrifyingly rigid nuns, loud city traffic, and the polio scare fed into my sensitivities. I would hyperventilate at night and faint often, and feared I would die and go to hell. Adult years were also difficult. At age seventeen, I was in nurses' training when students were used as a source of free labour. I was taught that I had a duty to care for others without thought to my own needs. Student-nursing days consisted of too much responsibility. As I did not train in a hospital where there was a medical school, student nurses were assigned medical-student responsibilities. At the end of three years, I regularly experienced panic and anxiety attacks. I married young and had three children by caesarean sections. After my first C section, I could not walk for weeks without severe pain. This was my first attack of FMS, but I was not diagnosed at that time. It would be thirty years later before I was told officially that I had FMS.

I began university at age thirty-two. I later divorced and became a single mother of three, experienced several months of being stalked, and eventually remarried a widower with two teenage children. By then my own children were teenagers. I pushed myself through a professional career working in a stressful university environment. This all served to reinforce my HSP tendencies. I did not handle conflict very well in my professional career. I avoided it as much as possible but would suffer excruciating pain as a result. Fibromyalgia attacks and chronic pain and fatigue were part of everyday life.

Since age forty-five when I began the process of self reflection, I have explored my own tendencies as a hard-driving, high-energy, caring-for-others-first type of woman. It has not been an easy task to change my way of being in the world, and the task is never complete; it is my life challenge. I can say with some degree of certainty that I have FMS because I was an HSP. I now can, most of the time, understand, if not control, the demon. I worked full time until retirement, and now I enjoy our small grandchildren. I rarely have anxiety attacks, and while the pain and fatigue are always present, they do not always overwhelm me as they once did. I do, though, have sleep disturbances and many physical inadequacies due mostly to the stiffness that accompanies fibromyalgia. Pain is always present. I will never recover completely from an easily aroused nervous system that has been over-stimulated throughout my lifetime.

I have done many things to search for relief of my symptoms. Most treatments have cost a great deal of money, but some are free. In the past, I have taken homeopathic medicine and, for sleep, amitriptyline, neither of which I continued for very long. I have regular massages and take several vitamins and supplements to boost my immune system.

I must exercise gently, or I suffer the next day. When not too vigorous, yoga has helped somewhat in the past. I have learned the techniques of "freeze frame," which I will describe fully in other chapters. Above all, I am privileged to have had an income which helped to pay for complementary therapies, although most have not been very successful. Chiropractors and massage therapists have helped greatly, but the effects are not as long lasting as I would have hoped, nonetheless they are effective and would have been more so had I begun these treatments at an earlier age; acupuncture has also not been very helpful. I have found that gently walking in a pool is very beneficial for me, as is walking in general.

In the next chapter, I will allow the voices of these women to be heard vividly as pain, fatigue, sleeplessness, and depression are discussed in more detail. With the exception of Mandy, all of the women believe that FMS was caused by their highly sensitive personalities. But what does that mean for us? Does this imply that we are our own worst enemies and should get a grip and control our minds over our bodies? Are we the culprits in all of this? Are we weaklings who give in to ourselves and our suffering? Have we victimized ourselves, and will my attempt to explain this highly sensitive nature and constantly over-aroused nervous system further re-victimize us? Needless to say, that is not my intent. There is a danger, however, that one could view my hypothesis as relating FMS to a psychosomatic disorder, which is not what I intend. That brings into question the whole concept of fibromyalgia as a real life every day challenge, but which could be erroneously perceived as a psychiatric illness. I prefer instead that those of us with fibromyalgia be perceived as having a gift of being able to sense things that others cannot, somewhat analogous to a canary in a coal mine. If the reader can keep this in mind, it will help with some of the unease caused by the theory that the condition is caused by oversensitivity, which some could label the fault of those who suffer from fibromyalgia.

3

Pain, Fatigue, Sleeplessness, and Often Depression

Living with Pain

What is it like to live with chronic pain? What do the women do when they cannot find relief from an invisible symptom—one that cannot be measured quantitatively, even though many scientists attempt to do so? Pain is a subjective experience that is contextually bound by age, race, gender, class, and culture, among many other factors. But what is that experience like on a day-to-day basis for the woman with FMS?

"Mostly, it occurs in my feet ... right down to the tips of my toes. I can almost tell you every bone and joint in my foot that I never knew I had, because it hurts," said Becky.

Sally, who lives in a different part of the country from Becky, spoke of waking her husband up in the middle of the night to ask him to take her to the hospital because she thought she was dying. She spoke of days where she hasn't "been able to get out of bed in the morning because of the pain I've been in."

Germaine says, "You live your life *always* with pain."

"It jumps around everywhere," describes Barbara. "Like an unwelcome guest, it never seems to leave."

The stories of the twenty women in this book are replete with serious debilitating pain so characteristic of FMS. Maddy is an extreme example; for her, the most serious symptom is the leg tetany for which she can find little relief. In his book about muscles, Thomas Griner[1] defines tetany as: "Hypertonic Spasm—The excessive, insidious, permanent contraction of a muscle caused by an accumulation of concentrated lactic acid." This is what Maddy experiences almost every night. In spite of heavy doses of pain medications, she still lives with what Griner would describe as permanent spasms. He writes that after twenty-five years of studying muscles, he can conclude that scientific medicine has overused drugs, that is, pharmaceutical treatments, for muscle pain relief in ways that are "unnecessarily dangerous" (p. xiii). Sometimes Maddy has full two leg tetany experiences that cannot be relieved immediately. Morphine and OxyContin are two of the heavy medications prescribed to her. These leg pains wake her at night. They can be compared to what we know as 'charley horses' that, for her, continue for several hours. While none of the rest of the women in this book suffer this extreme tetany of the legs, almost all of us had restless legs, generally after a bad day.

Needless to say, Maddy suffered great depression as a result of the pain, which left her totally debilitated. Over the years, she has been to many counsellors and therapists, most notably a certified activity therapist (osteopath) who does joint manipulation. However, it is the leg tetany that causes her the most pain. While we all suffer from pain in various parts of our body, restless legs is one of the most frustrating nervous-system aggravations.

Pellegrino[2] writes about restless leg syndrome and nocturnal myoclonus:

> These related conditions are most prominent at night. Restless leg syndrome causes leg cramps, especially in the calves, and an intense feeling of restlessness in the leg, that is not relieved until the individual moves the leg, as in walking around. Nocturnal myoclonus is involuntary jerking that occurs during sleep. A *neurologic* [my emphasis] mechanism, perhaps signals that don't get "turned off," may be responsible for both of these similar conditions.

But the pain of FMS is usually generalized to the whole body. How then to find relief? What are the women's experiences of living with pain? What is their subjective reality? If pain is neurological and not emanating from a particular localized area, why are we being treated for specific types of pain such as tetany or migraines with medications like antidepressants?

The physician Khalsa[3] writes that many doctors fail in their treatment of pain because they do not address its neurological aspects. As he says, "Chronic pain is in the brain." He points out that drugs, both painkillers and tranquillizers, are given as standard treatment for pain. Some of these, however, cause rebound pain. His advice is to nurture the nervous system to build neurological strength. Yet it is important to note that tranquillizers are given to many who suffer from FMS pain to help combat the accompanying depression.

"The specialist that I was seeing at the time couldn't get a handle on all the joint and muscle pain that I was having," explains Jane during our interview. "I went from ibuprofen to Advil (which is also ibuprofen) to Tylenol and to all those over-the-counter pain killers, and, you know, none of them worked. I see a psychiatrist [who] recommended I take Elavil in conjunction with these tablets which are Tryptan. I find them very helpful in terms of joint and muscle pain." Jane takes two 500-milligram tablets at night with 25 milligrams of Elavil, or amitriptyline.

The Canadian writer Marni Jackson, whose book on pain has become a valuable resource for those of us who live with this suffering, writes, "Accepting pain as something you must live with doesn't mean you shouldn't try everything from Pilates to Paxil to get rid of it. Giving in doesn't mean giving up."[3] None of us have given up; but our search is endless. A woman Jackson calls Alice describes her fibromyalgia as a "migraine of the body."

Jane considers the psychiatrist she is seeing for depression to be her best social support, in addition to the mood-altering drugs he prescribes. However, I wonder if he understands the source of her depression and its relationship to FMS. Do any health care providers understand? To what extent do mainstream psychiatrists understand psycho-neurological disorders and modes of intervention? More to the point, who does?

Vera says that her FMS began with pain in her elbows, which were sore to the touch. She describes her body as "hurty and achy." Anna says, "It's all over my body, you know, just pain throughout different places in my body." She takes Effexor for depression. When asked where she thinks depression comes from, she replies, "I think the pain is a lot of it, but I know it's ... know[ing] your limitations and not being able to handle the pain. It was the pain, you know, [that] got me, because I just couldn't seem to keep it in control." In fact, Anna had a nerve block on her back and then was given a back brace and told to walk eighty minutes each day. "I thought I was going to go to the nut house, it put me in so much pain." She said she cried most of those eighty minutes.

In a study conducted in the United States, the researcher Schaefer[4] interviewed eight women living with FMS. The women in her study described their pain as "bad, nagging, unremitting, agony, terrible, annoying, burning, and extreme." They described pain when it was at its worst, that is, during an acute attack. It has been my experience that acute attacks are episodic and occur a day or two after an unusual episode like stress, weather changes, or even the excitement of a happy occasion. Generally, they are short-lived, but the pain is often unbearable.

I can relate to Alice (in Jackson's book) who says that her acute flare-ups last three to five days. She talks about how hard winters are for her, and I also relate to that!

The FMS pain is ironically both chronic and acute. Chronic pain is what we live with every day; but a flare-up of acute pain is what I usually find more difficult. I am used to this nagging ache in most parts of my body, but I can be immobilized by an acute attack. Sometimes there are sharp stabbing pains like electric shocks, and I have to cry out. Other times I feel like I am coming on with the flu, and then an attack is not far off. The pain attacks one part of my body severely sometimes for days or sometimes just for minutes; it is totally unpredictable. It is not difficult to become depressed when the pain is unrelenting.

Leanne talks of her neck muscles as being so tight and heavy that she says it feels like a man's back and neck. It seems as though eventually all of us develop neck pain, which can be the most severe of all the pain. In my view, neck pain indicates that FMS is at its most severe and chronic stage, particularly when it radiates down the arm to the hands. I believe that after years of pain, we begin to anticipate it by habitually tightening the neck and shoulder muscles. While it may be true that certain kinds of pain are age dependent as discussed in chapter 1, I believe that the neck is one of the most common sites for FMS pain.

The study of pain and the view that "there are biological 'gates' that can be closed to shut off pain"[5] is not a new one, but research abounds with physiological explanations of general pain. It is not my intent to present the various theories of pain. I do not see much hope for FMS sufferers who have been part of research studies that attempt to quantify the qualitative aspects of pain. As I have previously mentioned, by its very nature, pain is contextually bound by gender, race, culture, class, ethnicity, age, and other factors—including the individuality of the person experiencing the pain and the unavailability of language to describe it.

Mandy said that black women in her community were not expected to voice pain and suffering. If she did, she was silenced by others. The "strong black woman" is expected to keep pain to herself and not act weak. Highly intuitive about and sensitive to these expected norms within her community, Mandy would not often complain to her friends and family. She suffered in silence.

Pain is a subjective experience. Tolerance to pain is also subjective and cannot be accurately quantified, and pain is expressed (or not) differently in specific circumstances. Those who experience it *may* have a particular "pain personality" such as that described by some researchers, but attempts to explore the intensity or kinds of pain associated with FMS are really not all that helpful. However, if my theory holds true that FMS symptoms evolve in the overly sensitive and intuitive person, it is more helpful to learn how to manage an over-aroused nervous system. I could explain the detailed intricacies of the nervous system, but the response from many with FMS would be, "So what?" What is the value of physiological theory, incomprehensible to those of us who are not experts in the area? We have pain; if it is caused by an over-stimulated nervous system, we need more help in understanding the psychosocial forces involved in the process. What can be done to help the nervous system diminish its responses to stimuli like chemicals, excitement, weather changes, poverty, stress, smells, sounds, and other external factors in our environment?

It is interesting to me that the 2003 CBC documentary on *The Nature of Things* with David Suzuki was entitled "A Disease Called Pain." In that presentation, Catherine Seton, a woman with fibromyalgia, gives the standard story about how her pain began after a car accident, and depression followed soon after. When she was finally diagnosed, she was told that her central nervous system and brain were chemically altered by the pain. Suzuki says that the dyad of the brain and central nervous system have emerged as active participants in the pain drama. However, several questions are not addressed:

- Why do women experience this phenomenon more frequently than men?

- Why do some women have whiplash (or other traumas) and not develop fibromyalgia?

- Why is chronic pain considered a *disease* entity?

- Why are the structural forces that impinge upon many women not considered to be precipitating factors?

The same questions are also relevant to those living with fatigue. We need to hear the voices of the women who are longing to have their stories told, who experience depression over the chronic nature of the condition and the lack of credibility paid to it within the health-care system. The personal is indeed political when it hits directly at our bodies.

Living with Fatigue

David Bell, a physician who is perceived to be an authority regarding fatigue, writes, "In terms of chronic fatigue, poor sleep is both a major cause and a major contributing factor."[6] It is therefore difficult to separate fatigue from sleep. It is also here that the distinction between CFS and FMS is not noticeable. Chronic fatigue is thought by some to be caused by

Epstein-Barr virus, but perhaps this particular virus may trigger chronic fatigue rather than cause it. But even then, this viral link is not without controversy. Still, there are tests that show that CFS sufferers have greater antibody levels than do those with FMS. Fibromyalgia, by contrast, does not reveal itself through any of the usual laboratory tests. Therein is the most perplexing difference between the two syndromes. Both claim fatigue as a major debilitating symptom, and this encompasses the greatest similarity. However, those with CFS do not *usually* have the same degree of pain as those with FMS. Wallace and Wallace (previously cited in chapter 1) state "that 20–70 percent of fibromyalgia patients have CFS, and 35–70 percent of those with CFS have fibromyalgia" (p. 50). This is another of those confusing statistics that fail to explain differences.

Though she describes her former self as high energy, Leanne now has to curtail her activities. "It makes you depressed because I mean, when you're … when you feel like your body is dying on you and your mind's alive, it's a hard thing to deal with when you don't have any physical proof that other people can see." She can no longer do some of the things she once enjoyed like dancing and gardening because of lack of strength due to fatigue.

Amy found the fatigue the most difficult. When asked which was worse, the pain or the fatigue, she replied:

> Oh! The fatigue. Probably because I was pretty badly injured when I was seventeen and so have pain from the athletic injuries and have learned to pretty much live with it. I know it's there, and I know what makes it worse, and I know some things can make it better, and I can pretty much get by—just say, "Fine. Deal with it." So had it just been the pain, I think I would have been able to handle it without too much effort, although it certainly was a different kind of pain; the pain is different. But not having the energy that I was accustomed to, that was really hard. Feeling like I didn't want to get up and move. I just wanted to be still. Then not be able to sleep. That, I think, is particularly cruel, this condition. You're so tired, and you go to bed, and you sleep like the dead for two hours, and then you're awake, and then

you sleep fitfully for the next six or seven hours. The fatigue is clearly the hardest thing.

A Swedish study[7] with fifty-eight women and three men with FMS found that the participants "referred to fatigue as the most disabling factor." It appears that pain is something one becomes used to living with, but fatigue interferes dramatically with activities of daily living. This is particularly the case as muscle strength is diminished. Even more maddening is that when the FMS person feels rather well and more energetic than usual on a particular day, she may overdo it and pay for it not usually on that day but, strangely, a day or two later, and the fatigue lasts for three to four days.

It is not possible to separate the pain from the fatigue because they are so closely related. Margot says, "If I walk too long, I won't feel any pain at the time, but the next day, I know that I've walked too far or pushed myself. The same as doing housework or any type of activity—I pay for it in pain the next day, or even sometimes two days later." It becomes a vicious circle as more pain initiates more fatigue. These women all know the price they have to pay for doing a little extra on the days they feel a bit better. They become depressed when they recognize that it is payback time for that little extra they have indulged in.

Mandy said, "I used to be a caterer, and I used to do in-home catering, and functions for three or four hundred people were nothing. [If] I did a dinner party for twelve, I was in bed for two days later. First day, flat out. Second day, start ... just starting to move around." This was very exhausting for her, and severe fatigue was the result. She said that she always weighed the pros and cons of doing certain things.

For each woman, fatigue ebbing from day to day coincided with the decisions made regarding the energy she had on that day. Diane said that even a shower resulted in fatigue, and afterward she had to lie down for thirty minutes to rest before dressing. For her, fatigue preceded pain. However, it was frustrating for all of us that we looked good and therefore were not considered to be feeling bad by family and friends. Fatigue, like pain, is invisible.

Some days I can hardly keep standing I am so exhausted. It hits all of a sudden, and wham! I can barely lift an arm and have to lie down. I know then I am about to have an acute flare-up. I often think I am about to come down with the flu.

Living with Sleeplessness

Varying degrees of sleeplessness accompany the pain and fatigue of FMS. How do we separate these main symptoms from one another? Which appears first? Do they all begin simultaneously? Any kind of reassembling and configuration of these main characteristics of FMS could elicit interesting questions. With one person, the limits of the nervous system could be pushed gradually toward chronic FMS, whereas with another person, a dramatic incident like a car accident could precipitate the condition. Therefore, is it possible that pain could be the first to rear its ugly head for some, and for others lack of sleep (because of child care, night duty, or too many home and work responsibilities) causes the syndrome?

In an American study [8] fifty women with FMS recorded their sleep quality for thirty days. A night of poor sleep resulted in a much more painful day, followed by another poor night's sleep. As in other reported incidences, pain and sleep appear interrelated, but fatigue also results from a poor night's sleep. Is it actually possible that sleep disorders come first?

I was a sleepwalker ever since I was a young child. I remember waking up curled in the deep porcelain kitchen sink when I was little. My earliest memories are of night terrors. Was the seed planted then for FMS? Was that the stage setting for what was to follow in later years? Elaine Aron writes that the hormone cortisol is present when someone is in a state of arousal, which then interferes with sleep. I must have a great deal of cortisol!

Diane spoke of being a light sleeper even prior to FMS. "But I don't know whether that was just because you're tuned into your kids." Many mothers turn into light sleepers, and I speculate that FMS could first exhibit itself when mothers listen for their babies during their own light sleeping periods at night.

Mandy and many others describe their sleep as "twilight sleep." "I can still hear everything that goes on," Mandy shares.

As mentioned previously Amy says, "Not to be able to sleep—that, I think, is particularly cruel, this condition. You're so tired, and you go to bed, and you sleep like the dead for two hours, and then you're awake, and then you sleep fitfully for the next six or seven hours." Amy describes how she feels after taking medication for her sleep disorder. "The side effects, the morning brain fuzziness … and literally it was …! I would take the normal dose, and I would be like a zombie."

Elavil did help, especially if I had a long holiday from it. Melatonin is better for me, though, as it has fewer side effects. I would rather take melatonin, as it is a more natural substance. I haven't taken Elavil for many years.

Clarke[9] writes how women and the elderly are "vulnerable to misprescribing." The use of allopathic medications for the sleep disorders of FMS is common. Equally as common are the side effects. Writing of the use of sleeping pills and antidepressants, Clarke points out that women "are more likely than males to use these psychoactive drugs by a 3:2 ratio." Even more disconcerting is the practice of prescribing sleeping pills for depression.[10]

Living with Depression

While all of the women experienced depression to a certain degree, it is difficult to know whether or not it was the result of pain, sleeplessness, or fatigue or if it was a primary depression.

"I'm on an antidepressant," Mandy says, "because they found that certain antidepressants help with the pain."

Becky explains, "I haven't had a decent sleep. I can't, because I have depression. I've been on Effexor and Alprazolam."

"This depression," Robyn describes, "it's clinical depression. It's very, very, very dangerous depression. It actually changes the way I think."

Mandy and Maddy have also experienced suicidal tendencies because of depression. The intensity of the depression varies greatly among all the women. It is obvious that the lack of a cure for FMS and the hopelessness of being slated for a lifetime of pain can bring about depression.

In a series of articles on depression in the *Globe and Mail*,[10] it is estimated that one in four women and one in eight men will suffer from depression. The dilemma is whether depression is the result of psychosocial and political conditions or biochemical imbalances or a combination of both. Nevertheless, women who have the many debilitating symptoms of FMS will no doubt also be depressed as they try to live with these ever-present challenges.

What can we conclude from this chapter? These women all experienced sleep disorders, fatigue, pain, and subsequent depression. Some described one symptom as more problematic than others. Nonetheless, it is difficult to separate one from the other as they all form an integral part of the same FMS demon. While some suffered from symptoms such as indigestion, irritable bowel, and other aggravating disturbances, it is still these four that together make up the main plot of the mysterious FMS tale and cause the most distress. When one component of the myriad of systems of the body is compromised, the others are affected as well. Most importantly, the symptoms cannot be viewed in isolation or expected to be cured or alleviated by standard Western medical treatment.

In chapter 4, I will discuss the gendered nature of FMS in detail. If it is primarily a woman's condition, what new knowledge can be deduced? What happens to diseases or syndromes when we attribute them to women only? Is there a FMS personality? Is this personality, that of the hyper-vigilant woman, contributing to a nervous system being in a constant state of arousal? If so, this is a societal problem and not merely an individual concern as mores and values regarding a woman's role continue to overburden many women.

4

Women and Fibromyalgia

Researchers who have only one idea and propound it over and over as truth can be vexing to many people. There is the possibility that I, too, may be seized by this idea of FMS and the highly or ultra-sensitive person, who can also be called a hyper-vigilant personality, to the extent I see no other explanation. There is no absolute certainty that I am right, yet I believe intuitively that those who have FMS have a very highly developed sensitivity, sense of responsibility, and perfectionism, and high energy is needed to fulfill those traits. Eventually, their nervous systems burn out, leading to physical ailments (muscle pain, fatigue, sleeplessness, night sweats, intestinal upsets, and others) and psychological pain (depression, brain fog, guilt, fear of being called a hypochondriac, and shame, to name a few[1]).

The psychologist responsible for the well-developed theory on highly hypersensitive persons, Elaine Aron, whose work I have discussed in chapter 1, has given me insights that have allowed me to view FMS from a new perspective. She does not discuss FMS or CFS, yet it appears to me that there is a strong relationship between them and HSP. This does not suggest that I agree with all of her tenets. I am not a psychologist, and the quantitative nature of the tools they use to measure certain kinds of qualitative traits is not my choice when it comes to quantifying qualitative characteristics such as depression or coping. I am uneasy with her view that HSP is usually inherited. As a sociologist, I tend to believe that hypersensitive people (in most cases women) are the product of their environments—that is, it is the nurture not the nature aspect that causes someone to become an HSP. In addition, in her book, she provides quizzes to assess various symptoms, and when a person scores a particular number on a quiz, she or he is then pigeonholed into a specific classification. In my view, this kind of data analysis is too arbitrary. Women's natures are multifaceted. A person's feelings can change frequently and responses to such quiz questions are not always consistent from day to day, perhaps even from hour to hour. Consequently, responses could vary frequently; emotions and feelings are not static. Rather, it is the gestalt that I am seeking.

While there are those in the scientific community who believe that unless phenomena can be quantified, data are not relevant, I believe that it is imperative to present experiential information in the form of narratives. The natures of many mysterious conditions like FMS are too complex to unravel with mere statistics. In spite of this shortcoming of attempting to quantify qualitative characteristics, Aron does not use self-administered questionnaires to the extent of most psychologists. *The Highly Sensitive Person* is, in my view, a breakthrough on issues of sensitivities, but it is the relationship of hypersensitivity to FMS that for me is the most intriguing.

Others have suggested that those with FMS are suffering from posttraumatic stress syndrome or are ultra-sensitive or hyper-vigilant personality types.[2] These people are thought to be overly in tune with their surroundings, intuitive, and not well protected emotionally. Being in a state of hyper-arousal begins in the nervous system but eventually compromises other systems of the entire body.

However, most of these theories to which I subscribe, lack a critical analysis regarding gender, race, class, culture, sexual orientation, and ethnicity. They are socially constructed as though these kinds of personalities are genetic. It follows, therefore, while unspoken, that those theorists believe that since women are more prone to FMS, women have innate characteristics. This kind of "essentializing" of women's nature is damaging to the woman who wants to be taken seriously. It negates the influence of women's ways of being in the world.

There are more questions than answers with regard to how a person can be perceived to be a highly sensitive person. In any one culture, being sensitive may be perceived differently, as may be the case within different cultural and socioeconomic classes. These issues must be teased out before a person can label herself as a highly sensitive person, such as Mandy did when asked if she perceived that there were more life difficulties with black women who had FMS than with white women. Wallace and Wallace suggest that, in fact, there are fewer black people than Caucasian people with FMS (previously cited). This may be because more white people have access to medical resources or because there are race differences regarding reporting of pain. It is likely that black women meeting racism within the health-care system are less likely to divulge their pain to the predominantly white physicians with whom they come in contact.

":[In the] black race," Mandy begins, "the women are the most dominant figure when it comes to child rearing and home management. And, you know, to say that you're in pain or whatever is a sign of weakness, and that's what we were always taught. You don't cry, you don't show pain, you don't do all these things because it means that you are very weak. And to be weak was more of a disgrace than admitting that you were in any kind of agony. To be a strong black woman meant to hide pain from others and to consider others before herself."

Yet Mandy suffered quietly. It is possible to speculate that if one has constraints on her life like racism, heterosexism, or poverty, to name a few, then FMS is more likely to develop but less likely to be reported. The research about this aspect of FMS is nonexistent.

It is also possible that many of the people who develop FMS might, in fact, be experiencing posttraumatic stress disorder (PTSD)[2] as well. This is most likely with the women in this study who said they began the journey to a FMS diagnosis following a car accident or a hysterectomy, both of which are physically and psychologically traumatic to the body. While I find the idea that secondary FMS is precipitated (not caused) by an accident, injury, or severe illness somewhat compelling, I cannot accept the view that physical trauma survivors are the only ones most likely to develop FMS. It may be that highly sensitive persons who suffer serious traumas have, in fact, been pushed past their limits and are then in states of over-arousal of their nervous systems. However, this PTSD episode may be secondary to a lifetime of over-stimulation of the nervous system.

The question to address now is whether or not there is a personality-prone FMS person who is predominantly female. While I am very uneasy about suggesting that women are more prone to FMS because of their socially induced sensitive characteristics, it is impossible to negate the gendered nature (as well as the statistics) of FMS and CFS. I doubt that FMS is only physiologically based or that it is passed on from mothers to their children through their genes. Rather, I believe that it is the result of the ways in which women are living their lives in a society that expects more of them in terms of sensitivity, round-the-clock vigilance, and caring for the emotional and physical needs of others. In short, constructing gender psychosocially and politically jeopardizes women's health. While it can be argued that women more than men are usually (but not exclusively) conditioned to be more sensitive to the needs of others, in my view the ultra sensitive person has developed this trait to such an extent that it becomes dominant in her personality. This eventually affects her autonomic peripheral nervous system (ANS) so that the *parasympathetic* ANS (the slowing-down subdivision) cannot function effectively, leaving the body in a constant state of hyper-vigilance and over-arousal. This results in the *sympathetic* ANS (the accelerator) telling the body to work harder and faster and to remain under stress. This imbalance, therefore, results in hyper-arousal, sleep disorders, fatigue, exhausted muscles, and subsequent pain. Is this problem more common in a woman because of her biology, or is it specific to an individual woman or to her genes or to an entire society? This remains the important question.

More broadly, Finkler[3] attempting to discern why women generally become sick more often than men, develops the concept of "life's lesions." She writes, "I hypothesize that the concept of life's lesions is significant in comprehending morbidity cross culturally and across class lines." She maintains that we must attend to the cultural and social contexts of women's experiences throughout the life cycle because they produce more non-life-threatening sicknesses in women than in men. Still, in the case of FMS, the psychosocial focus has been on symptoms such as pain and fatigue (the effects) and how to cope with them rather than on exploring in-depth the causes of FMS that may be more socially based. Theories on coping, which are structural-functional in nature, suggest that if that person does not cope, then the individual is at fault for being unable to adjust to the pressures of society, followed by instruments for coping. The women in this study did not use this language, describing themselves instead with voices different from the medical paradigm.

Now I present the voices of the women themselves speaking of their own personalities and why I interpret them as highly sensitive persons.

AMY: I think there are personality types that either put themselves in positions where they're constantly testing their limits, and that can get translated into episodic stress.

While she was saying this, I wondered if that is quite accurate. Maybe another way of framing this is that life's circumstances place these women in situations of frequent stress either through a lifetime of sexism, racism, hetero-sexism, economic insecurity, or abuse of various kinds. Then perhaps the nervous system kicks in as usual and hyper-arousal results so that even the activities of daily living become problematic.

AMY: I think there may also be accidents of fate.

Yes, that fits! Fate as in to whom one is born and where and other life circumstances.

AMY: I was just talking to a colleague two days ago who has a very good friend who was sexually assaulted two years ago and has finally begun just recently to begin to sort of pull her life back together after this horrific experience and then suddenly developed symptoms which were inexplicable, and she's been diagnosed with fibromyalgia. And her rheumatologist told her that she, the rheumatologist, believes there is growing evidence that women who have had that kind of life-disintegrating stress may be more vulnerable to develop fibromyalgia. And you gotta wonder. I think it all boils down to neurochemistry, and there's no way that I can say that that kind of event doesn't profoundly alter the neurochemistry balance of the nervous system, alter it over a long period of time.

May be more vulnerable? That sounds right. This is the ultra-sensitive person whose nervous system is in a state of constant hyper-arousal.

Interestingly, we women described ourselves as high-energy people who had to change our lifestyles after being diagnosed. This kind of almost frenetic lifetime hyperactivity was discussed as a "superwoman" type of person.

JEAN: I used to be very energetic to the point that I wondered what was wrong with me to have this strong drive to be on the go constantly. I rarely sat down. After working hard all day, I would fill every evening with activities or sports and housework. Small things bothered me a lot, and I became very anxious and irritated over things over which I had no control. I felt I couldn't waste a minute on such unimportant tasks because I needed to do a perfect job on the things that were so important to me. I would get agitated very easily.

Aron writes about HSPs who are "out too much in the world." She suggests that those of us who are out too much are not protective of our bodies and, hence, abuse them. She talks of the out-too-much person as one who is that way even with her leisure activities. The body craves down time and rest from over-stimulation.

I remember being asked by a massage therapist to notice how quickly I did things, even brushing my teeth. "Do you brush them in a hurry?" he asked of me. My answer was yes!

AMY: [I] always [had] enormous amounts of energy, always [had] enough energy to do whatever I want[ed] to do and to push as hard as I wanted or needed to push.

ROBYN: Very much an A personality. Prior to all this happening, I'd wake up at six o'clock in the morning. I'd play racquetball. I'd lift weights. I'd go to work. I'd work twelve-hour days. I was an aggressive worker. I'd cycle. I was constantly active, always on the go.

MANDY: How do I describe myself? Outgoing, a person who's always on the go. High, oh, very high-energy-type person. And they've done research on that, and they said that most people who have fibromyalgia are high-energy personalities.

High energy is, in essence, an arousal of the nervous system, which Aron describes as "anything that wakes up the nervous system, gets its attention, makes the nerves fire off another round of the little electrical charges that they carry."[4] Conversely, Aron's definition of "in too much" (is more of a recluse) might appear to be antithetical to the high-energy person. Or is it?

BECKY: You know, I really think there is a mind/body connection with it. Because the people who I talk to who have it seem to be people who are very, I don't know, aware of their bodies. They are people that tend to ... I don't know, think a lot, take great concern with other people. I don't know how to explain it, but they're ... they seem to be thinkers, feelers, sometimes more of a quiet personality, but not always, but they're more in tune with themselves.

Although FMS women are in tune with what is happening with their own bodies, we do not stop and care for ourselves first.

LESA: I'm a dancer, and I've always been told to rely heavily on my imagination, which is what I do for a living. I get myself all bound up in this, and I imagine whole scenarios, and I go through them to the bitter end in my head.

But being aware of her own body through movement did not mean that she thought of caring for herself before caring for others. Aron suggests that HSPs have rich, complex inner lives. Lesa exemplifies this by saying that she often imagines herself in other people's positions.

While all of us experience self talk, I believe that the HSP does more of this, creating real or imagined conflicts or insensitivities, as she embodies all that is going on around her. Lesa does not like confrontation or conflict and describes herself as a worrier. Worriers often imagine the worst scenarios, allowing self talk to dominate their responses to stimuli. Worriers wonder if they are doing enough for others.

I'm a worrier. My parents are worriers. Small events became disasters. Anticipating and fearing the worst was a way of life for me. So I go to extremes to be super organized so that I can be prepared for the worst; but, of course, the worrying has not helped at all. In fact, I feel miserable after an episode of worrying. Catastrophic thinking is a way of life in my family of origin. Optimism does not come easily to me.

SALLY: I've always been, since I was a little girl. I've always been a worrier.

LESA: Well, I know I worry a lot about things. But I keep things in; I don't like to show that I'm worried or upset. People think I'm very laid back, but inside I actually just don't like to cause problems, so I just keep quiet.

Worry is the anticipation of fearful events, imagined or real. In her workbook for HSPs, Aron writes:

> We HSPs, probably more than other people, carry the effects of many, many moments of overstimulation, stress, fear, and trauma. Where do we carry them? In ourselves, of course—our organisms, our bodies, and our brains included. And sometimes we have been so sensitive we have had to cut ourselves off from our sensations in those overstimulating moments to keep from being overwhelmed. If others were the cause of our being overwhelmed, we may have used our sensitivity to tune into what they wanted, hoping to appease them, instead of attending to what we needed. Indeed, sometimes our very survival as infants and children depended on our talent for tuning in to what others wanted. Later, that effort to please and appease others may have driven us in our work or other achievements.[5]

BARBARA: Do you care for other people's needs before your own?

JANE: Usually, which has got me into trouble relationship wise.

BARBARA: Because you don't get your own needs met, I bet.

JANE: No. No. I seldom do, to be honest with you. And even, you know, with my friends and my family, I find that even if I'm tired and I'm in my bed, if a friend or a family need me to take their sick child to the doctor or, you know … anything. I will get out of my bed, and I will go and do that for them … I can't help it.

MICHELLE: I don't usually take a lot of time out to take care of myself. But prior to, you know, just go and go, whatever someone else needed, regardless of how I felt.

While it was obvious from our conversations that we all tended to take care of the needs of others before ourselves, the situation has changed dramatically, and there was another kind of psychological pain occurring now because of our inability to do as we did before.

ANNA: Sad, because I worry about the relationship with the rest of the family, that they think I'm not doing enough.

LOUISE: Now, all the time that I've been off work, I've never slept during the day because I'm not supposed to. It took me months to realize that I was off work, and I could bloody well sleep if I wanted to. I felt guilty. Even for all those months after I left work, I would feel guilty.

Where did I get this view that the mother must be self-sacrificing? I usually think of my children's needs before my own even now that they're adults. I often worry that I am not doing enough for my children, who are much stronger than I am. I've done it to myself by not placing boundaries around what I can do and what I can't. I am not "supermum!" I don't usually make my own needs known; it's what we women do. My own mother did it; so do I. I know it's time for me, but old habits die hard. We're martyrs for others' needs.

Along with the guilt about not doing even more for others is a sense of shame. The tendency to hide FMS from others is voiced frequently.

ROBYN: I'm very self-conscious about my illness. So I actually pulled myself in about five years ago.

MANDY: Bad days I have. I hibernate, too, because I don't want anybody to see me in that condition. And, like, none of my friends are, or outside of my immediate family, have ever seen me in a bad day. I don't talk about my pain to people, unless I know that they are either a pain sufferer or in the health system. I only talk to people who are in my support group about the pain because other people don't understand. Even my husband, he says he understands, but really he doesn't.

Only recently did I talk about FMS with the people I worked with daily. In fact, many of my friends don't even know I have it. I rarely (if ever) even tell my children or close friends how badly I feel and how much pain I am in or how fatigued I am. Because it is invisible, people think I am stronger than I really am. Why bother others?

BECKY: The people think I either come up with these illnesses or that I'm looking to be sick because every six months there's something else wrong with me. And I get to the point where I'm not telling anybody because they'll think I'm out of my mind having so many illnesses when they're all fine.

LEANNE: (I'd) like to get away from the guilt, get away from the self negativity.

What can be concluded from the voices of women who fail to speak openly of FMS except to health professionals and a select few others? The answer is very complex, having to do with societal views of the woman as a caretaker for others to the exclusion of her own needs. Some women fear they will be considered hypochondriacs, and others fail to speak of their conditions because of guilt or shame or because they do not want to burden others. The ways in which the women speak of their lives and the language they use to describe how they try to hide their pain from others is very telling. All the women caringly want to keep their problems away from others. As Becky says, "There's no point in telling them because they get concerned." These women feel guilt at not being able to perform at peak but simultaneously anticipate that by telling they will inflict pain upon others.

Is FMS a disability? If so, it largely remains invisible, unless, like half of the participants, the sufferers use a cane at some point. I believe FMS is a disability. Most of the women I spoke with are not able to work outside the home, although all want to do so, and all have to curtail activities of daily living to some degree. But as people with an invisible disability, except for the two women with MS, they are not accorded the role of people with diminished capacities.

What then can be gleaned from all this? It is probable that women with FMS have un-reconciled psychological pain that has become manifested as physical pain through constant stimulation of the automatic nervous system. Rather than labelling a woman as a specific personality type, I would prefer instead that there be opposite knowledge developed that focused on societal conditions impinging upon women. If more women are in hypervigilant[6] states or always on duty to serve others before looking after their own needs, it is likely that the number of those with FMS will continue to increase. Health care for women must take into account societal expectations. Jennifer Howard[7] writes:

> True gender analysis has to consider the social roles and power that we all live with as women and men, by virtue of our gender, as well as the impact these gendered roles and behaviours have on our health. For most people, gender is as invisible, and as important, as the air we breathe. Unless an analysis that compares how and why women and men are affected differently by policy is applied to programs designed to improve health, these initiatives will likely fail for both women and men.

Furthermore, if we continue to focus on the symptoms of FMS to the exclusion of its political and psychosocial causes, we are merely applying a Band-Aid.

In chapter 5, I will discuss the environmental triggers that precipitate flare-ups as well as the kinds of support that are needed in times of acute episodes. The women's voices will be heard once more as they discuss the meaning of social supports in their lives.

5

Triggers, Attacks, and Supports: Women Speak Out

Speaking out about challenges that are invisible to others and often considered nonexistent to health-care providers can be devastating. In fact, the language to describe the experiences of FMS patients is even problematic. It is sometimes difficult for doctors and patients to determine the nature of pain and fatigue. Is the person who is suffering in a chronic, or an acute flare-up stage? Or even more confusing, are the symptoms caused by something other than fibromyalgia?

Flare-ups often occur a day or two after a stimulating event such as excitement or stress, weather changes, or eating certain foods. Conversely, an acute flare—up can occur a day or two before a weather change. The person with FMS must always be keenly aware of what has precipitated an acute attack. The price that has to be paid for the stimulation that occurs following any kind of unusual episode is an acute phase of FMS, consisting of severe pain and extreme psychological disquiet, which seriously affect sleep and fatigue. It is generally greater pain and fatigue than the chronic type.

Following a remission from that acute attack, which could last several days, is the kind of chronic but often less severe pain, fatigue, and sleep disturbance.

Those who experience FMS face another dilemma when deciphering what comes first: pain, fatigue, sleeplessness, or depression. This chapter will discuss triggers for acute attacks—these shared experiences of pain, fatigue, sleeplessness, and/or depression as precipitated by environmental and psychological stressors—and the kinds of support that the women receive from family and friends. I also include some information about the difficulties of living with an invisible condition that brings about guilt and shame.

Flare-ups, Triggers, and Attacks

For me, the flare-ups are generally caused by stress, excitement, or weather. The summer brings humidity; at that time, I seem to ache constantly. When the humidity is high, my pain level increases dramatically. Winter cold, fog, rain, mould, and even indoor heating systems can be triggers. Nova Scotia is not a good place to be any season.

BECKY: Weather changes! And it seems it doesn't matter what it's changing to. For a while, I thought it was just when it was wet, and it would be really bad … the pain and the burning. My hands are really bad right now. We had a week of a lot of rain there; my hands were in terrible shape, and my feet. And then when it got really cold, I thought, good, this is going to be a little better. And it's slightly better. During the [weather] change, it got worse, and then when it's just stayed cold now, it has calmed down a fair bit; it's not as bad as it was.

VERA: I find that I have an average of two days at least every couple of weeks that, no matter what's going on, I'm feeling very emotional, very down, achy. The weather certainly plays a part with me as well. The first two years we were south in the wintertime, I never had an ache or a pain. As soon as I came home, I could hardly crawl in and out of the door.

MANDY: I know that climate changes and that pressure in the atmospheric conditions make it worse. I know that cold and damp make it worse.

ROBYN: I died last winter. Dampness. Dampness affects my pain. That humidity! I couldn't believe it. I normally don't mind the heat. [Robyn switches from winter to summer as she speaks of dampness]. I just … I just … this has been the worst summer I've ever had.

LEANNE: Sometimes I don't know what triggers [the flare-ups] because there's so many allergies that I seem to have that I don't know what's triggering what these days. Certain times of the year, it's worse—fall—and then I'll have a couple of months where it's okay.

KERRY: I hate [humidity]. I hate it! I don't like, I hate it! Can't stand [the cold]. I hate being cold.

Summers in Nova Scotia are dreadful with so much humidity. I suffer great pain and fatigue from the dampness. Winters aren't all that great either, especially with severe cold. In fact, only autumn is relatively pain free, except if it's a rainy autumn! Yet while on sabbatical on the west coast in both Victoria, British Columbia, and then later in Vancouver, British Columbia, both moist climate cities, I felt wonderful. Is it stress combined with weather? David, a friend and a scientist, says that while he has traveled often to many places, including cities that are by the sea such as Victoria and Vancouver, he has never seen the kind of green and silver mould that exists on trees in Nova Scotia. Can this be a precipitating factor too?

SALLY: It's worse in the winter because I find it damper in the winter and there tends to be more rain and snow in the winter than at other times.

While most of the women speak of weather conditions triggering attacks, all speak of stress and excitement as also being a big factor. Peculiarly, the pain and fatigue are not immediate. One might expect that these symptoms would occur almost immediately after a stressful or exciting event. But it is almost as if the muscles are using up what little reserves they have, and, finally, after a day or two, the pain and fatigue set in.

JANE: I love music, and I love to dance, and I'm usually the life of the party. And I mean that. But at the end of the night, I pay for it. By the time I leave there, and my body has run out of steam, I can hardly walk up the stairs, you know, to get home, because my feet are just swollen, you know. And, of course, the next day, don't look for me, you know, because I'm in bed. You know, my body has to recuperate. And you just learn to live with that part of it because you know that if you push yourself that next day it, it's just not … you, you can't function.

MICHELLE: I find that most of the time I'm really not that interested in going anywhere. Like, I find that the thought of the energy that I have to exert to get ready to go somewhere seems like more than what the trip is worth to me. To spend the time getting ready to go out for, you know, an hour or two hours, it just hardly seems worth it, you know, because not only will I be tired from taking the time to get ready, but I'll be tired being out, so then tomorrow's going to be a really bad day.

ANNA: Depending on how hard I drove myself, it may even be tomorrow [when the pain appears] as well. I found when I was doing [dental] hygiene it would take at least a day and a half to almost get over it, from working as a hygienist. The pain would take that long to go away.

Support Systems

What then can people who suffer from these devastating symptoms expect from others, particularly considering that most women are not comfortable asking for assistance? Many of the women spoke of the kinds of support they needed when experiencing a FMS attack. Some received help from spouses, family, or friends, while others often felt they did not receive any help from anyone, especially during these acute phases.

LOUISE: My husband is terrific. I mean, when I quit work … maybe three weeks later, he took a week off work to be with me … to do all the housecleaning, all the housework, vacuuming and all—everything. He is wonderful. He is wonderful. And you know, I mean, because I wake up five, six times a night groaning, because I would, you know, groan out loud. It would wake him up. He was the one who had to get up in the morning to go to work. Did he complain? No.

I scare my partner when I groan aloud with severe pain. But he is the only one that I will allow to hear me. With others, I suffer quietly, yet I dislike being the martyr. Once I terrified my parents during an acute attack when I cried out in severe pain. I felt so badly afterward.

DIANE: My husband has been very good about rubbing my feet.

KERRY: Now, I do have a very dear friend; he lives in Montreal. And not that he knew a whole lot about it when we met. He knew that I was sick, and he's been very supportive from day one. That's my biggest support system. But just talking to my friends in general? No, that's not something [that gives support]. My mother's been very supportive, very supportive.

Some women found a psychiatrist to be the most helpful. For example, one said, "I see a psychiatrist, and I have been seeing him for the last seven years approximately because my doctor, my GP, he really doesn't seem to know a whole lot about fibromyalgia, and I don't really get the feeling that he's all that interested in learning about it."

Not all women found comfort in spouses, family, psychiatrists, or friends.

ANNA: My husband is the one that ends up cleaning [the house] because it bothers him. Compared to what he used to do and especially where I'm working part time. I think the assumption is there that I should be able to do some of this stuff.

LEANNE: My partner is [supportive], but he still doesn't understand because he's a scientist-kind of person, and I guess he's figuring, like, maybe I'm not doing enough to make the doctors hear what I'm trying to say. And friends, yes, [they're supportive], but it's like I have a few friends who are, but it's sporadic. And, like, it's very hard because, you know, it's a hard one, because how much do you ask your friends to do? You know, how much can you expect and that kind of thing? So there are times when I think that we could ask for help, but we don't.

Accompanying this resistance to speak of pain and fatigue to others is the fear of being labelled a hypochondriac and complainer. When labelled as someone who complains frequently, shame, guilt, and depression set in.

Depression

MANDY: You don't cry; you don't show pain. You don't do all these things because it means that you are very weak. And to be weak was more of a disgrace than admitting you were in any kind of agony.

Mandy was describing the issue of being a black woman not showing pain in her community, but it was common for all the women—black or white—to keep it to themselves and then feel depressed.

LEANNE: There's always the concern that should you go for counselling or anything that someone could easily label you with some illness because you're depressed over a chronic illness which they don't understand, or they don't consider the fact of what that does to people.

ROBYN: I was like a hypochondriac; I was after doctor after doctor after doctor to help me. I felt so desperate.

Robyn takes medication for depression. The discourse around being labelled a hypochondriac was fearful and shameful because it is pejorative and often attributed to women. The end result is chronic depression. She says she has no support whatsoever.

BECKY: Talking to you, I just felt totally redeemed for once. I could have cried to think that, my God, this is real, and I'm not a nut case, and I'm not just a wimp too weak to take whatever everybody else does.

Feeling legitimated allows the women to release their self-depreciating self-images and causes an upswing in mood. Candace tells about visiting a psychic who told her she had fibromyalgia. Many times, she visited her family doctor, who, after many visits, told her she did not have fibromyalgia. However, after the psychic had "diagnosed" her, she became convinced that she did have FMS. Finally, her physician concurred, and she felt legitimated. Her support was the psychic rather than the family doctor.

CANDACE: I'd say I've got the burning between my shoulder blades when I am on the flights [as a flight attendant] and when I'm pushing and pulling carts, and in the chest, the pain, and the chest and the soreness in the chest if I press on my chest in the bones and stuff … chest (pain).

Burning between the shoulders is so common. This happens to me frequently. It also rotates to the chest. Wallace and Wallace discuss costochondritis, a common and scary irritation causing chest pain. In fact, I once saw a surgeon for this very condition, frightened that it was breast cancer.

Real or Imagined? Keeping It Hidden Can Contribute to Depression.

Many of the women initially thought it was their imaginations that produced the FMS symptoms and that they were not, in fact, real. Many so-called women's conditions have been dismissed as being "all in her head" by doctors and psychiatrists. The women's experiences are consistent with this dismissive history.[1]

MADDY: Because I wrote it off as psychological and something I needed to work out and handle myself, [I] never credited it as something physical. In fact, when I brought it up, I said it may be all in my head, but the symptomology is making my body such that I can't get through the days, much less work.

Others spoke of the fact that it was invisible, and therefore discounted.

KERRY: Well, that's the thing—well, even with EI, you know. We talked about it one day at the clinic. There was a guy there, and he said, "What's so frustrating? People look at you and say you don't look sick. Because it's on the inside, they don't see it." And grant you, when I really get a bad day, I do look sick. I get really dark under here; my color goes grey.

Most of the women spoke of the pain of hiding their conditions.

SALLY: Because of my attitude towards it, I don't show people that I have it. Like, I don't, or very seldom, I will admit that I'm in pain. And it's very seldom that someone will look at me and say, "Oh, you look like you're in pain today."

It was not just the invisibility that prevented the women from speaking of their pain or fatigue, but rather it was because they did not want to burden others. This ties in with my view that many women who embrace the commonly held view that women should suffer in silence are hesitant to speak about their symptoms. This is especially salient in conditions that cause pain but cannot be categorized by professionals as more than invisible, mysterious conditions. The highly sensitive person does not want to cause a problem for others. It is not her habit to seek care. Rather, she is the caregiver. These feelings of guilt, shame,[2] and disappointment because we cannot perform in our usual highly efficient manner (as before FMS) produce anger that seems to rule our lives. However, the anger turns inward and manifests as depression. Not being believed, hiding the challenges of everyday living, and worrying about the reaction of others can easily cause depression.

The majority of the women I spoke with expressed their ongoing challenge with depression. Michelle says, "Anything that the doctor has ever given me for depression has taken me further into it." Anna takes Effexor for her depression. I asked from where she thought her depression originated.

ANNA: I think it's a combination. I think the pain is a lot of it, but it's your limitations and not being able to handle the pain. And just things start to bother you, just your personality type. And, I don't know, I always figured it was the pain that, you know, got me because I just couldn't seem to keep it in control. It just kept getting worse and bothering me more.

KERRY: You go through this depression mode. Like this week, I've been going through depression. And Sunday I was really depressed. I'm ironing, crying, ironing, crying.

MADDY: EMDR [eye movement desensitization reprocessing] is a therapeutic technique [developed along with others, primarily in the wake of the Vietnam War] for dealing with trauma and depression. The hypnotist? Another route to the early trauma which I cannot recall cognitively through memory, etc. I also want to talk to him about using some of the newer antidepressants if need be.

Doing much better on the painkillers and antidepressant (Celexa—latest version of Prozac) think it is helping, at least I am not blubbering all over the place. Just started last week so should have an idea of how well it works within a couple of weeks.

From the interviews, I found that dealing with pain, fatigue, sleep disturbances, and depression is often an overwhelming task. But none of us could say whether pain, fatigue, depression, or sleeplessness came first. However, there is some degree of relief for many people. In the next chapter, I will discuss some of the ways in which the women deal with FMS on a daily basis. Specifically, I will discuss the kinds of symptomatic treatments that were employed in order to live as fully as possible.

6

Treatments But No Cure: What Can Be Done?

For women who suffer daily, it is not easy to sort through the various strategies and treatments that may or may not alleviate some of the more troublesome symptoms. The process generally involves a wide-ranging search for temporary relief to enhance one's quality of life while recognizing that currently there is not a cure for FMS. For many women, there are relatively few available choices, especially as cost is a big factor, and most complementary treatments, which could perhaps provide some relief, are not covered by health-care plans. For the more economically privileged, trial and error is the only means of finding out what might work for them. A particular modality may work for a while and then become ineffective. New symptoms develop, leading to another set of treatments that could be in conflict with an existing regime. The search for effective, albeit often temporary, relief of symptoms is long and arduous. In this chapter, I will highlight the kinds of treatments that are most commonly used by the women in this study.

In spite of many difficulties, all of the women had strategies that they believed helped them somewhat. These strategies encompassed such varied complementary modalities as practicing imaging, having a massage, or using Western allopathic medications for pain relief and sleep difficulties.

Most of the women in this book found some degree of relief with medications for sleep, mainly antidepressants. Candace, Jean, Maddy, Amy, Mandy, Anna, Margot, Vera, Jane, Lesa, Germaine, Sally, and I have sometimes taken Elavil (amitriptyline), the most commonly prescribed drug for FMS, although not all of us continued to take it for long periods of time. This antidepressant, in a mild form, has been somewhat successful in helping with sleep and pain for people with FMS.[1] A newer drug, Neurontin (Novo-Gabapentin), is becoming increasingly popular. The side effects from Elavil are few and usually short-lived, except for weight gain and next-day grogginess. However, most of the women did not stay on this medication for too long because it became less effective after a period of time.

I had been on Elavil for longer than all the other women in this book—almost ten years. I had gained thirty pounds from taking it. I usually only took ten milligrams, and without it I would be in a twilight sleep. Even with it, I did not have a long, restful sleep. Sometimes I took twenty milligrams, but I hated doing that, as I then needed a higher dose just to maintain that level of sleep. I have been off of it now for over ten years. Now I find that melatonin is as effective, without the side effects.

CANDACE: [Elavil] was helping some. But it was the weight that I was gaining, so much weight. And, I mean, and [living] alone trying to get around, I was very uncomfortable. So then I went and asked [my doctor], and then she changed it; she gave me some Inovane. And that seemed to work out okay. It seems to me my body … I go for a while, things work really well, and then they don't work so good. I have a very high tolerance to medication. And, like, I could take medication probably that somebody else would put them right out on their, you know, out on the couch, and me, I'd be walking and talking.

BECKY: With the fibromyalgia, now, over the past year or two, I haven't had a decent sleep. I can't, because I have depression. I've been on Effexor and Alprazolam and take Alprazolam at bedtime, which helps me to go right to sleep, which is, again, unusual for me to go to sleep that quickly; it wasn't natural, but now I do. But I wake, it feels like every ten minutes, but I'd say I look at the clock about every half hour or hour before three and six in the morning.

That is the same as what I experience. I fall asleep quickly (usually) for about two hours; then I awake usually every hour or so until I get up. It is nonrestorative sleep and feels like being half awake and half asleep. Everyone I speak with and all the research I've read about state that this twilight sleep is a main characteristic of this condition.

But not all the women take allopathic (prescription) medications to help with sleep. Many of those who did take them found the side effects of weight gain and sluggishness the next day too distressing to continue with their usage. Only one of us had tried a natural herb for sleeping.

VERA: Well, since I've been off the Elavil, I've started on nerve ones, valerian. Now I've been taking two of these since last Thursday, and I find that I've slept pretty good with them.

Kerry spoke of a friend with FMS who took melatonin, which is naturally produced in the body, for sleep. It is evident that there are few medications that are effective for sleep difficulties associated with FMS over the long term.[2] Goldberg suggests herbal or natural supplements can be effective. He writes, "Helpful here are melatonin (3 mg) before bedtime; valerian herbal extract (150–300 mg) taken thirty minutes before bedtime; or GABA (gamma aminobutyric acid, an amino acid derivative), taken at 200–400 mg, thirty minutes before bedtime."[3] I personally have not tried any except melatonin, an alternative to the conventional medications, and I have not heard anyone speak of them as being effective over the long term.

Sleep deprivation is very problematic, as "brain fog" seems to be common following a sleep-disturbed night. Williamson describes how people explain this as "a feeling that clouds the brain, that there is a fog surrounding them that keeps them from really being in the world."[4]

While sleep disturbances cause brain fog, it is clear that fatigue is equally significant after a night of sleeplessness. Kerry speaks of the exhaustion she felt prior to going to the Environmental Centre. At the centre, she would take a sauna to detoxify, and she also learned a technique known as "freeze frame."[5] She describes this as a series of five-minute exercises that help her alter her stress level. She tells of trying to work while feeling so badly. "It was like having the flu every day without the full-blown flu—just totally exhausted." She would put her feet up on her desk at work because she couldn't "push no more."

Kerry explains that she is currently getting better. "For about a year, I was doing the intravenous therapy [at the centre] during which they will put minerals and vitamins into you intravenously." She also speaks of eating for her blood type, which helped her considerably.[6] While Kerry is doing relatively well because of her contact with the Environmental Centre, she has found that going back to work has aggravated her condition once again. She praised the centre for the vitamin and mineral therapy and the sauna sessions, which, she says, cause her to perspire and decrease her toxicity.

At the Environmental Health Centre, I was shown this "freeze frame" technique by Dr. Fox. It is a computerized program somewhat like biofeedback with which patients are treated as a form of therapy to control stress in their lives. It is a technique developed at the Institute of HeartMath and measures pulse-rate variability. It is used to determine whether a person can bring his or her autonomic nervous system into balance. In my view FMS should be treated as though it was caused by over-stimulation of the nervous system, using certain techniques like freeze frame to settle the body and mind. Kerry also thinks so and practices this at home. It can be done at home or anywhere without a computer and is an excellent way to reduce other conditions too, like fast heart rate and even hypertension.

It is significant that none of the women in this study were able to do much about fatigue. While all of us took at least one vitamin and/or mineral supplement, none of us have found relief from fatigue if we had a greater-than-usual sleep disturbance the previous night. I therefore speculate that it is sleep loss and sleep deprivation that cause fatigue and pain and the subsequent depression. Allopathic medications are not available to cure the sleep problem; these medications only provide temporary relief, and the search for pain relief is ongoing. In addition, overusing allopathic medications can lead to addiction as most require an increase in dosage over time.

BECKY: It has been almost a year now since I have been using magnetic products to ease the pain, aches, burning, and sleeplessness. I wear a magnetic necklace, bracelet, and earring every day and have dramatically reduced the pain in my neck, hands, and jaws. I also wear magnetic insoles in my shoes, and they stopped the pain in my feet. Now I sleep on a magnetic mattress and pillow and under a far-infrared quilt. The effect has been that I drift off to sleep easily and in a relaxed state without medication.

Some of the therapies for pain relief that we women have undertaken include:

- Various massage therapies … I am fortunate in that I have massages regularly.

- Chiropractic manipulation … I have regular chiropractic adjustments.

- Osteopathy and meditation

- EMDR(a psychotherapeutic technique developed along with others, primarily in the wake of the Vietnam War, for dealing with trauma and depression, which I have not tried)

- Magnetic therapy

- Hypnotism

- Homeopathy and naturopathy … I have taken homeopathic drops, but they proved to be ineffective for me.

- Herbs … I have taken various herbs but they too proved to be ineffective for me.

- Acupuncture and electrotherapy … I have found a bit of temporary relief results from Synaptic 2000, which is stronger than a TENS machine. It is a device that modulates natural neurotransmitters through cutaneous stimulation, which induces the body to release serotonin, a neurochemical that influences pain and mood.

- Stretching ... A good water-aerobics program that encompasses stretching is often effective and I have engaged in this practice in the past.

- Walking, particularly in a pool ... my favourite.

- Recumbent stationary biking and yoga ... I tried both in my younger days but due to the on-going stiffness that comes with aging and prolonged FMS I am unable to do so now.

- Therapeutic touch and Jin Shin Jyutsu ... which I found to be soothing.

These therapies for pain can be considered 'complementary' to the usual over-the-counter pain medications. This is congruent with the findings in a study by Schaefer[7] who found that "all the women used complementary approaches to supplement care, including herbs, homeopathy, acupuncture, relaxation tapes, hot showers, and massage." It is difficult though to equate massages, hot showers and relaxation tapes with alternative therapies or even complementary therapies as many in society use these forms of relaxation frequently in their daily lives.

It is increasingly obvious that many women are seeking alternative strategies to Western-style medicine. Is this because therapists (like naturopaths or homeopaths) more than other health professionals are able to spend more time listening to their clients or because the women have given up hope that Western medicine can help conditions that are sometimes vague or invisible to the usual kinds of medical testing?

Jean, who has tried many forms of complementary therapies, gave advice to others with FMS:

Try as many of the techniques as possible to deal with the disease [sic]. Exercise, stretch, rest, try alternatives such as massage, electrotherapy, acupuncture or whatever is possible.

Several of the above-mentioned modalities are not exactly complementary or alternative (with the possible exception of acupuncture, which has even now become mainstream) but rather substitutes or good health practices, like stretching and exercise. Generally, complementary or alternative therapies are considered to be those in the form of herbs or homeopathic solutions. While these are often hotly debated in terms of efficacy, with the pros and cons of alternative or complementary modalities taking on a life of their own, the move to 'holism' has nonetheless been dramatic of late.

"I miss my airjet massage tub," Maddy wrote when she was away from her home. "But I have been swimming and doing [abdominal] exercises regularly in the pool." Airjet tubs or exercises cannot be considered to be alternate therapies in this instance. Yet, an airjet tub can be considered an adjunct to pain medication, thereby labelling it complementary. The debates in this arena are both fascinating and somewhat confusing. What exactly is a complementary or alternative therapy?

The trend of late has been to consider nutrition a major factor in the "defective" bodies of those with FMS and CFS,[8] and some researchers believe that microbes "emit a continuous stream of inflammatory chemicals resistant to antibiotics," a situation that can be resolved by taking supplements for making glutathione. Whether or not vitamins, minerals and other forms of supplements are considered to be complementary or not is also debatable.

I no longer use the 'holistic' approaches such as homeopathy or naturopathy because they have not helped me in the past. Yet, there are advocates of both therapies who will find some degree of relief and are no longer trusting of Western medicine. However, many people cannot afford them and they do not cure FMS, as far as I know, and they often provide only temporary relief. Most importantly, a holistic approach, like Western medicine in general, focuses only on the individual, not on a societal responsibility for the role of women in our communities. If relief is available through complementary herbs and homeopathic drops, then why are they available only to the economically privileged or to those who sacrifice other essentials in order to pay for them? Has this recent turn to what has been considered to be a more natural way of healing only become a panacea for other psychosocial problems facing women in this turbulent era? These are difficult questions to explore. But most of us with FMS have, whenever possible, tried everything we can afford to obtain relief from our condition. We do not simply rely on others to cure us.

McKee[9] writes about how dangerous it can be when the burden of blame for health problems (particularly on women, in the case of FMS) is placed on those who suffer rather than on societal obligations and responsibilities.

The health-care system and its institutions and lack of resources and services are often barriers to good health. Most people do have some control over their own lives, and there are a few inexpensive ways to alleviate some of the suffering. These include meditation, stretching, and walking, which have been found to be effective for settling the nervous system. But we must acknowledge that living in pain and with fatigue can result in a lack of motivation. Those who are in very difficult economic situations can hardly be advised to buy expensive walking shoes or get to an exercise club. It is important to point out that there needs to be a concerted personal effort for those with chronic conditions such as FMS, which comes often at great personal cost to the individual and economic cost to society. But there also needs to be a social commitment to eliminate those conditions that militate against a good quality of life, particularly for women who are suffering economically.

How then is it possible for a midlife woman to turn her life around at a time when she believes, as one woman in my interviews, that her body has burned out? If women with chronic fatigue are too exhausted to undertake exercise regimes, too worried about finances, too depressed to try meditation, too sleep-deprived to concentrate, or experience pain on a daily basis, then how can they expect to have the reserves for this added effort when their internal and external environments are already over burdened? It is likely that any energy she has will be spent in caring for others before caring for her own self.

Midlife women who can no longer work either at home or outside the home and/or are economically disadvantaged may also be experiencing physiological changes from perimenopause, menopause, or postmenopause. How much extra effort can be expected of them? In the next chapter, I present some answers to these questions about menopausal women and FMS, since it appears that this is when the most dramatic crises occur. Most likely, however, I will be left with even more questions. In particular, how does a mid-life, hypersensitive woman undo the learning that she has taken a lifetime to achieve? And, very significantly, does FMS actually improve with old age after the older woman has realized she can no longer be the caregiver she once was? Or does she always remain with her highly tuned sense of the feelings and needs of others?

7

Midlife, Menopause, and Fibromyalgia

As has been stated in earlier chapters, the symptoms of FMS include over-whelming fatigue, nervousness, brain fog (described as memory lapses), joint and muscle pains, anxiety, chemical sensitivities, sleep disorders, indigestion, irritable bowel and depression. Yet ironically, these same symptoms also sound like ailments associated with menopause. The Canadian sociologist Janine O'Leary Cobb first wrote of women's experiences of menopause in the 1980s as a result of her own menopausal experiences.[1] In her newsletter, *A Friend Indeed*, she and her contributors cite about fifty symptoms of menopause. One volume of this newsletter, which is regularly sent to hundreds of midlife women, was specifically about menopause and fibromyalgia.[2] In her book *Understanding Menopause*,[1] O'Leary Cobb writes that fibromyalgia aches and pains do differ from menopausal pains, which are usually restricted to one or two joints. Nonetheless, the similarities are striking. In this chapter, I discuss the complex issues facing midlife women with FMS who are perimenopausal, menopausal, or postmenopausal. The similarities between menopause and FMS are often confusing, and I speculate about how difficult it is for a woman to sort through each stage of menopause in order to situate herself as an aging woman with the chronic condition of FMS.

Simone de Beauvoir in *The Second Sex*[3] uses the terms "lived experiences" or "concrete situations" of women's lives. The experiences of menopause, hysterectomies, and hormone replacement therapy are examples of the concrete situations of many of the women in this study. They are gender specific and affect the myriad of challenges that are faced on a daily basis by women living with FMS.

Hysterectomies and the Midlife Woman

Why are hysterectomies so common among midlife women? Why is there so little research on the impact of this surgery on women? These serious questions cannot be easily answered, but they are especially relevant to the topic of FMS as I speculate about whether or not a hysterectomy can precipitate the condition.

Women who have had a hysterectomy and have FMS face a triple burden. Sandwiched between the older and younger generations, they often face both home and occupational dilemmas, while simultaneously experiencing hormonal fluctuations of menopause.

"Why don't you have a hysterectomy?" the female doctor asked me at thirty-five after I experienced heavy menstrual bleeding. "You don't need a uterus anymore."

I'm happy that I insisted on keeping it, as maybe my FMS would be even more debilitating. What I really needed was quiet, calmness, and respite from overstimulation. "Why would anyone want to have unnecessary surgery?" I asked her. Did the women in this study who had hysterectomies suffer more FMS as a result?

Of the twenty women in this study, there were eight who had a hysterectomy,[4] a large number indeed. Did the FMS develop before or after the hysterectomy or simultaneously with menopause?

BECKY: Well, I think [FMS] happened for me after my hysterectomy that I had in 1993. It took me a full year to feel anything near myself again, and so that would have been 1994. I've noticed since then, within that next six months, I started having a lot of hand and wrist pain and just never regained the strength and stamina that I had before the surgery. I blamed it on all kinds of things—on estrogen levels and all those kinds of things.

LOUISE: I had a hysterectomy when I was quite young, but I still had my ovaries. And I think I went through menopause fairly early, you know, the hot flashes, and so I've been taking estrogen—hormone replacement therapy—for quite a number of years, so I don't have a problem with that. But the prednisone [which was prescribed for myalgia, which, to be accurate, is not considered to be quite the same as fibromyalgia] does affect your hormone balance. Because then I remember going for blood tests and I thought I'm going to tick off [on the requisition form] FSH [follicular stimulating hormone] just because I feel something. So, sure enough, [the doctor] said, "Whoa! You're post-menopausal." "Ah," I said, "well, so I'll increase my estrogen then, won't I?" See, I could tell.

For Louise, the difficulty was sorting through the fibromyalgia and menopause issues and dealing with the use of estrogen replacement along with other pain medication and prednisone. As a midlife woman, she was now in a quandary as to which condition she should be dealing with more intensely.

In conjunction with the confusion, Louise did not know precisely when FMS developed, whether it developed simultaneously with or independently from the hysterectomy. She did, however, notice a decrease in her energy, which she believed would increase with more estrogen.[5] Were her health concerns FMS, menopause, or both?

VERA: Yes, I was [in menopause]. I had gone through a forced hysterectomy when I was forty-two, and so it was very hard for me to know when menopause was coming on, and I was going through some of the [FMS] symptoms [at the time of developing FMS after a car accident and whiplash].

Vera was also on a transdermal patch for hormone replacement to ease menopausal symptoms. It was not possible for her to know whether or not the patch helped. It was confusing for her to figure out if it was the hysterectomy, menopause, FMS, or even the effects of the car accident causing her many ailments. These life situations in a self-proclaimed highly sensitive person could easily result in hyper-arousal of the autonomic nervous system. She was caring for an ailing mother and working in a situation where she intuitively perceived herself as redundant. It had taken until her middle years when her reserves were depleted and menopause had begun before she began asking questions about her life.

Kerry also had a hysterectomy within the past five years.

KERRY: I was going through flashes. [Barbara: Are you in menopause?] No, that's why I wasn't quite sure. But now when I get these flashes ... see, I used to think, mm, hot flashes, but now I don't think so. And then when I read up on fibromyalgia, that is one of the symptoms.

The confusion that was present for Kerry and the other seven women who had gone through hysterectomies, was related to whether or not the flashes were the result of their hysterectomy and subsequent menopause, FMS, or midlife concerns.

Doctors are also puzzled by the effects of hysterectomies and menopause on FMS, and further blood testing of the women's hormone levels (FSH) is usually done. But it is also difficult for women who did not have hysterectomies and were in menopause. Mandy said that she was in menopause when FMS began, and it was difficult separating the two. Her hot and cold flashes have subsided somewhat with hormone replacement therapy but not entirely. She had grave concerns about taking HRT.

I did not take hormone replacement therapy. So many of the women wondered about whether or not they should be taking estrogen, or hormone replacement therapy. Why are there so many difficult choices for women? We feel as though our bodies and minds are no longer friends to us, yet we don't know where to turn to begin an even keel.

LESA: At forty, I had my womb, ovaries, and cervix removed. All of it. So I have been on hormone medication because I wasn't ready [for menopause].

Lesa developed FMS soon after her hysterectomy. Is she experiencing menopause simultaneously with FMS? Since menopause is a natural process, I am not presenting it as a disease to be contended with as one reaches a certain age. Whether because of accelerated stress in midlife (often coined as the sandwich generation), economic insecurities, or other predisposing psychosocial factors, it is likely that the women who did have hysterectomies experienced one more assault to an already overstimulated nervous system. It is little wonder that given all of their life stresses, particularly sleep disorders, all of the women in this study, even those who did not have a hysterectomy, spoke of brain fog as common (no doubt due to the sleep difficulties[6]).

Brain Fog

One of the many common frustrations of menopause is brain fog, or memory distortion.[7] This symptom is also common in FMS. Lesa said, "It happens at the weirdest times. I could be walking down the street ... and I just lose a sense of reality or something. I forget where I am, who I am, just momentarily." Sally, who did not have a hysterectomy, began menopause early at forty-three and was on hormone replacement therapy. She described her lack of concentration due to FMS and/or menopause as "brain farts." The question to consider is whether or not this lightheadedness or fogginess is due to menopause, FMS, aging, or simply lack of restful sleep.

ANNA: I don't know whether they're scattered [thoughts], or I find that you go to pick something out of your brain, and the screen's empty.

JANE: But a good day for me still means that sometimes my words might come out backwards, you know, something like that. And maybe I might forget to turn down the street [where] I should have turned.

VERA: I think my memory's gone though, too. I really do think that [FMS] affected my memory. Now I don't know whether that's menopause or whether it's aging or the fibromyalgia thing or not.

SALLY: You just get so muddled. Or you forget things. You'll go to do something and it's not like ... oh ... it's not like someone normal will forget something and stop and think about it, and it'll come to them. On some days, you just can't see the reality for the fog that's in front of your face. That's just the impression I get that I'm in this great big fog, and I'm just kind of looking for things, and I'm never going to find them.

MICHELLE: There's times that it scares me, because sometimes I'll be driving and all of a sudden ... how'd I get here?

JANE: I'm not really looking forward to going [to the Environmental Centre]. I'm not. Simply because, I'll tell you why. They send you this big package with probably a thirty-page questionnaire. That's a deterrent right there for me. I don't have the attention span or the concentration level enough to sit down and fill out a thirty-page questionnaire. It would probably take me a year to do it. You know. So ...

Menopause and FMS

It was interesting to note that most of the women experienced FMS at about the same time as perimenopause, menopause, or postmenopause.. Germaine said that FMS occurred two years after menopause. Although Robyn developed pain in her thirties, she was tested for hormone levels and found not to be menopausal. However, after menopause at age forty-eight, she had full-blown FMS. Jean has difficulties deciding if she is menopausal or not; hormonal tests have shown two different results. It is likely, however, that she is postmenopausal because women with multiple sclerosis tend to go through menopause earlier than the average woman.[9] Yet when she was fifty and at least perimenopausal, she was finally diagnosed as having FMS.

CANDACE: She [the naturopathic doctor] was treating me at times for hormones. I was to her in the summer, and I got really discouraged, and I just didn't bother going back. At first, she was treating me with hormones, and then she was treating me for the fibromyalgia. Then I didn't go for a while, and I went back, and then she said, "Well, I'll give you this for now, and then we'll go back. If this doesn't work, we'll go back to the hormones." But like I said, I got discouraged and paying all kinds of money out, and I didn't feel any different. [Barbara: Are you in menopause?] They've never told me that, no. Premenopausal, I guess.

Robyn was two years postmenopause and taking hormone replacements.

ROBYN: I take hormones. Yeah. I'm not happy with my hormones. I'd like to get, I'd love to be able to afford to go into an independent lab and have all my hormones checked.

JANE: I patch every day. Yeah, that's how I get my estrogen.

Nurse researchers McElmurry and Huddleston,[10] writing about the lived experience of menopausal women and the patterns found in menopausal studies, indicate that "much of the research has focused on the signs and symptoms of menopause that could be relieved by HRT [hormone replacement therapy] rather than on the menopausal woman and her experiences." The same could be true of FMS. Others have said that menopause causes a woman to be considered to be in a "deviant" role.[11] Once again, the same can be said of FMS. O'Leary Cobb[12] writes more hopefully, "We may also be witnessing a backlash against the biomedical model of menopause." If that is indeed so, then maybe we will also see a turn away from the biomedical model of FMS.

Like menopause, FMS research consists mainly of sample studies of white women. There is a scarcity of data specifically related to different ethnic groups and women from other countries, but this is slowly changing.[13]

Both FMS and menopause are gender issues, and until we have data from women in countries outside of North America and Europe, we will continue to make faulty assumptions that are ageist, racist, and classist about midlife women. Just over twenty years have passed since the term "involutional melancholia" (depression caused by menopause) was dropped from the *Diagnostic and Statistical Manual of Mental Disorders* (DSM), the bible of psychiatric diseases. Are the depression of FMS and the depression of menopause experienced in the same way? More research is still needed in these often intersecting areas of concern for women.

Germaine Greer[14] writes about menopause as a time when women become "less self-sacrificing," "more preoccupied," "less accessible," "less predictable," or "less biddable." She writes, "Mothers and wives are, in my experience, seldom self-centered to begin with, especially by comparison with both their husbands and their children. The perception of a less obliging female as more self-centered seems to carry part of the resentment felt by family members if the mothering function ceases to be the focus of a woman's life." It would seem then that the woman who is or has experienced menopause at the same time as FMS is at a crossroads in her life.

Can she give up the usual feeling that she must be all things to all people and instead consider her own needs first? Can she mother herself? Can she find ways to calm an overstimulated nervous system that has been in a constant state of arousal from all the physiological, social, and psychological pressures? And again the question arises: when she finally becomes senior, does her FMS fade along with the menopause symptoms? Does FMS diminish with old age?

I am now a senior citizen. I have retired from a stressful job. My kids are on their own. I have a wonderful spouse. I am privileged. Yes! The acute fibromyalgia attacks have subsided somewhat, especially as I am able to get away from the Nova Scotia climate when attacks become intolerable. The research is not available yet, but I do wonder if with older age fibromyalgia does lessen in intensity? Aha! Is it because I've entered a time of life when the needs of others are not as intensely seen to?

In the next chapter, I will discuss how the women kept on with their difficult lives and still maintained courage and some degree of hopefulness.

8

Women Spirit

This chapter is about perimenopausal, menopausal, and postmenopausal women who live with FMS and yet know how to survive with the constancy of hypersensitivity toward, for, and about others. Joanna Frueh[1] writes, "Ancient peoples believed that postmenopausal women retained their menstrual blood, called "wiseblood." Wiseblood made wise women. Here are some of the words of the wise women and their optimistic "women spirit," which strives to sense, feel, and meet the needs of others. It is the kind of spirit that keeps the world afloat, but at a great personal cost. While most women are socialized to take care of the physical and affective needs of others, I believe that those with FMS live within a framework where this intuitive energy is exaggerated. These are women who are in tune with their environments, like the canary in the coal mine, to such an extent that they should be revered for their talents. But at what cost to them?

Socialization differs from one culture to another. Similarly, there are race and class differences. Poor women, women with disabilities, and women of color face double, triple, or quadruple jeopardies of sexism, ableism, racism, and/or classism (Some women will face additional discrimination if they are not heterosexual.) While there are huge differences in women's lives, those who have FMS and possibly CFS (as it is becoming increasingly difficult to separate the two) have taken on the real or imagined slights, hurts, pains, and even joys of others and themselves to such an extreme that they have developed ultrasensitivity and heightened vulnerability to the entire environment. In spite of this, they keep surviving regardless of their physical and mental pain and often find inner strength because of their determination. There were many strategies they used to help themselves.

KERRY: Well, see, I try to keep my spirits. I've been, I've kept my spirits up all through this, anyway. At the beginning, I didn't. But I'm an outgoing person anyway, so I try not to let that destroy me, because no matter what stress I've had in my life, I still try to keep a smile. Actually, that was brought to my attention last because I helped somebody, and I was depressed because I was [unable to do as much as she wanted to]. You go through this depression mode.

GERMAINE: I think if you go home and sit down, your pain is there, and you just think about your pain. I think if you get active but know your limits, learn how far you can go, and when you get tired, just take it easy. Take a book and read or ... or do something. Play cards.

ROBYN: I meditate, normally, twenty minutes twice a day. That really, it helps me calm down. I like it for other reasons though. Other things that I do for myself, when I can, and when I can push myself to do them, is exercise. And I think exercise, quite frankly, as hard as it is for us to do, and I'm in and out of it, is probably the best thing we can do.

Robyn and several others kept on exercising with sheer determination because they did not want to be seen as laggards. They were afraid of being thought of as lazy, and they wanted to feel hopeful.

LEANNE: I'm optimistic that I will get bouts of energy where I can try to force [health professionals] to investigate further, push them to do what I feel is their job, to give me fairer health care to the best of their ability.

MICHELLE: I'd like to think I'd get better. But I don't know. I guess, for me, if I could just not get worse and just kind of feel, you know, have even a couple of days a week that I feel really well. At this point, I'd kind of be content with that, I think, you know.

SALLY: I don't like to let anything get the better of me. And I figure that I'm better than this fibromyalgia. And so sometimes I feel if I just ignore it, it's going to go away. It doesn't. Other days, I feel I can just get out there and get my muscles moving, and it's going to work; and sometimes that does work. And when I was swimming every day, I felt better, and I had very ... I had a lot less incidences when I was in pain.

VERA: It'll pass. That's the only nice part about the whole thing. It seems like it, if you have two or three bad days, eventually you're going to get the good days.

LESA: I think so [upon being asked if she thought that there was hope for the future]. I think there probably is [a cure for FMS]. And I think it's a matter of deciding, like, I recently quit smoking. And I think it's a matter of, of will for everything.

MANDY: No [she does not have hope of recovery]. I've learned to ... as I said, it took me a long time, but I learned to live with the fact that there is life after pain, or life with pain. There is life with pain; it's just that you have to learn to regulate and control that life. [Barbara: You don't give up at all, do you?] No, I just keep on going regardless of, I know that if, that's the only way I can function, because I've always functioned that way. But see, for me the hopelessness is a very dangerous position for me to be in because it leads to suicidal thoughts, and it leads to ... because I am all or nothing. So this is the way it's going to be, and if I dare give up, then what's the point of being here?

KERRY: Having fibromyalgia. Well, whoa. I don't know, but you've got to hang in there, and you've got to keep that chin up. I mean, it's very frustrating. I mean, we get our down, we get our down days; there's a lot of days I cry every day. That's with the mood swings. But you've got to keep that chin up, you know, and just ... and with me I just feel like, okay, life does go on. I have to live. I have a five-year-old son. I have to do things, so I have to keep going.

While it can be seen that these women have a degree of optimism, there is little doubt that following a diagnosis of FMS, a change in lifestyle is essential. This can be very unsettling and frustrating for the midlife woman who has spent her life anticipating the needs of and feeling intensely about others often at the expense of herself. The knowledge that she is unable to be the superwoman of the past and that she must now tend to her own needs often results in feelings of hopelessness, uncertainty, and fear of letting others down. It does not get rid of her highly developed intuitive nature. However, these women cannot be portrayed as helpless victims. It is evident from these anecdotes that the women display real courage and spirit in the face of adversity.

A concern for the highly sensitive person is how to adjust to a new life-style without feeling negative about herself and losing her spirit. How does this woman who has extra intuitive perceptions forsake past behaviours and focus on herself? This woman spirit has sustained a compassionate and caring person. How does she learn to reorganize her life and her perspective now that her past ways of interacting with the world have been somewhat curtailed? For all the women, it was the wearying characteristic of being a "sensing, intuiting, thinking, and feeling" person, as Aron calls most HSPs,[2] that does not change while she attends to her own needs.

It is clear what these women are saying: somehow they will carry on *despite* the inability to do so in the same fashion as before. Their words led me to believe that they would keep on going despite their wish to continue to be there for others as they have always been. How does one continue—in spite of pain, fatigue, sleeplessness, and depression—to express some degree of optimism for a lifestyle that is unfamiliar? I believe that the idea of "keeping the chin up" is valiant in the face of uncertainty over a diagnosis of FMS, the lack of credibility among health professionals regarding a sufferer's plight, and the necessity to live a different kind of life without further compromising one's own health. These women seem to have found some degree of understanding that there are reasons to be somewhat optimistic in spite of their daily challenges. At the same time, they realize that change is inevitable.

What happens to a woman in her childhood is integral to the patterns she establishes in later life, and that it is difficult, but not impossible, to change in midlife. I do not have much detailed information about the childhood intimacy issues that affected each and every one of the women in this book. However, I do know enough to say that, despite their different backgrounds, these women faced exaggerated societal and familial expectations. In fact, it is probably more so for the black women who, no doubt, have had even more expectations placed upon them as the stalwart gender holding the fabric of their communities together.[3] I do not have data that suggest that FMS or CFS is more common among women in the black community, but I would venture to speculate that it is highly likely, even though Wallace and Wallace suggest that the reverse is the case. It is likely that it is more underreported among the black population. It seems impossible for a black woman to feel the extreme pain or discomfort of others of her race and to feel hypersensitivity for those others and not suffer negative repercussions from that intuitive, psychological sensitivity leading to an over arousal of the nervous system.

The issues related to the hypersensitive person cannot be separated from the idea of caring. However, in writing about the HSP, Aron does not concisely take her thesis to that level of analysis. My view is that the HSP is so attuned to the needs of others and how the moods and feelings of others affect her that she develops an "overcaring,"[4] overly responsible, overly conscientious, and overly perfectionist mode of exhibiting her concerns. It is as if she wants to take away the pain of others by absorbing it as her own. She is willing to sacrifice her own health for the well-being of others around her. As early as 1988, Gordon[5] wrote that young girls think and care for others before caring for themselves. They become highly conscientious, a trait that Aron suggests is integral to the HSP.

My son was married by a lake, and after the ceremony, the justice of the peace asked them quietly to point out the most responsible person (of about a hundred guests) to care for the marriage certificate. Their faces turned to me, from a distance, and they beckoned to me to take the document and keep it safe. At the time, I was happy to be singled out as the most responsible person among the group. I was always conscientious to an extreme. It has not been an easy trait. As the elder of two children, my mother always bragged that I was the responsible and strong one in the family, and that was why I became a nurse. But there, I experienced the pain of my patients, and it was not a healthy environment for me. Sometimes I feel like I have been caring for others all my life. A women's studies graduate student once told me that I was "like a mother to us all." I don't want to mother the world. Stop! Let me off!

But how does one change a lifetime habit? It's the body that has finally forced the change.

DIANE: I no longer know the pace I should be at; tasks are done at a much slower pace. My children are grown and don't even live nearby, so I have only myself and husband to think about. At one time, I was one of those supermoms; now I'm a very boring person! But that's life! I think I've just depressed myself while rereading this [e-mail] message.... Guess I'm trying to tell you that living with fibromyalgia and MS for years sure changes a person—you're never what you used to be, and it changes your thinking and approach to things.

BECKY: I feel a certain measure of peace because I have decided what's important to me in my life and really, for me, that is me and my family. And so the rat race can go on; I'm not going to participate in the rat race. If the rat race gets beyond me, and they want me out, I'll be out, and I'll find something else to do.

LOUISE: Am I trying to fulfill my life with these imaginary responsibilities because I can't do "bugger all?" I don't know.

Just as there should not be any essential concept of woman in any society, there is no attempt to "essentialize" women in this book (that is, assuming all women have similar experiences). While we have similar health issues, we have different ways of dealing with the changes that FMS brings to our lives. We are not all alike, in spite of our FMS ultra-sensitivity and over-stimulated nervous systems.

Diane realizes that she must do things at a much slower pace, while Becky re-evaluates her priorities. Louise asks if she is trying to imagine more and more house tasks to be done in an effort to fulfill herself. By contrast, Kerry keeps pushing herself, trying to put on a positive public face. Aron says that it is difficult for the HSP to complain even if it is legitimate.[6] In addition to not complaining, many women are undemanding.

KERRY: I have to keep going. And like, there's things, like there's times that you do have to push just a little bit harder, and, like I said, with the walking—that's something that's recommended the moment you go to the Environmental Clinic [Centre]. They recommend some form of exercise. So I try to do that as much as I possibly can. The days that I don't, that I don't feel good, I don't go. But I try, and I always try to keep a smile.

Jane Aronson[7] writes about change that she thinks "could relieve women of the privately borne pressure to be dutiful and undemanding and permit them, rather, to give and receive care by choice in keeping with the particular nature of their wishes and capacities; foster in older women a sense of entitlement and confidence in articulating their needs without shame; and, in younger women, foster a sense of entitlement to pursue their own interests and development without a sense of guilt and inadequacy in relation to others."

I'm embarrassed when I have to ask others for a favour. I feel so inadequate. I find myself apologizing for asking. I'd rather do it myself even if it hurts physically to do so. It's much easier to say I feel fine when asked how I am. I don't believe that anyone really wants to know, except other HSPs, and I don't want to burden them anymore than they are already. I hate being thought of as a complainer. But the great part about getting older is asking people to do things for me and not feeling as guilty as I once did.

BECKY: I mean, I've told a couple of friends at church, and they're concerned and they'll say, "How are you doing today?" And it's almost like I can't be bothered to answer because they don't want to listen to the long explanation, and it's no better, and there's no point in telling them that because they get concerned. And they want to know, "Well, what exactly is wrong?" And then I, you know, I can't say I've got this pain, that pain. So I just say, "Oh, you know, about the same." So it's okay because they don't see it either. They'll say, "You look good today; you must be feeling better," and I just go along with it and say, "Oh, yeah, I'm not too bad today." It's just too much to get into, and they don't understand it.

It appears to me, then, that the midlife woman living with FMS is overwhelmed and over-stimulated, caught in the struggle to maintain a sense of control over her own well-being while keeping most of her problems to herself. She may be caring for children, grandchildren, aging parents, a partner, or friends and processing their needs and feelings to the exclusion of her own. As the result of a heightened sensitivity to others—not only in her own personal realm but in the entire sphere of her being—her own body and mind has suffered. Yet at the same time, she has developed guilt and shame from what she believes are her own inadequacies. Whether or not her sensitivities are appropriately intuited is not even an issue, because whatever the woman perceives as real actually becomes her own reality. Nevertheless, in spite of all these challenges, these women have strength, a sense of hope, and the courage to get up every day and push forward.

However, the problems of FMS are made even more difficult when sufferers are forced to convince others that their condition even exists. What happens when this syndrome is thought by those in powerful positions to be nonexistent and long-term disability becomes not a right but an issue to be hard fought? Even more troublesome is: what if my theory is correct and used by those in a position of power to further victimize women? These are the questions I will address in the next chapter.

9

Disability: Struggling To Be Believed/Struggling For Economic Security

On May 12, 2000, for the second year in a row, Mayor Pennington of Lumberton, North Carolina, declared a "Fibromyalgia Awareness Day." He stated, "Whereas, if employers would support their employees with FM by making changes to the work environment, persons with FM could continue to function at work and not have to file for disability."[1] While this is a rare and progressive approach, one for which the mayor should be praised, in this chapter I present divergent views. These are ones I find difficult to write about because I am so intimately involved with the topic. Not all people, particularly physicians, are as open-minded and insightful as Mayor Pennington. Many are harsh, and their actions (intentional or not) demean a large segment of the FMS population. Some people, though, are sympathetic and helpful as they can be. Still, others take a more neutral and cautious approach to FMS as a disability.

Discussing the Canadian situation, McCain, Cameron, and Kennedy[2] write:

> At present, fibromyalgia is a significant cause of long-term disability and is often the subject of prolonged litigation in Canadian civil courts. As such, it presents a major challenge, not only for the diagnosing physician but also for the 3rd party insurers and lawyers who are involved in the struggle for fairness in compensation and disability claims. Problems unique to fibromyalgia arise primarily because of its

perceived subjective nature, uncertain duration, and natural history, as well as substantial long-term costs.

The question about whether or not FMS is an actual disability continues to be ongoing. Arguments both for and against the diagnosis of FMS as a disability are numerous. It is useful to briefly discuss the concept of disability, particularly as it is a political issue.

Moss[3] argues that we need to move away from the notion that disability is about a medicalized condition of an individual and instead focus on the ways society itself is organized. He defines disability as "the disadvantage or restriction of activity caused by a contemporary social organization which takes no account of people who have physical impairments and thus excludes them from the mainstream of social activities." Not only are people with invisible disabilities often excluded from social activities, but they are also often unable to work. They then suffer great economic hardships because either they are not believed (as is often the case of FMS and CFS) or their employers are not supportive regarding long-term disability. With one exception, the women in this book were forced to stop work or take a leave of absence, and those without spouses were particularly concerned about finances.

Financial Difficulties

Robyn speaks of being bankrupt. "I'm used to earning, the ten years prior to [FMS], I was used to earning anywhere between $60,000 to $70,000 a year." Now she finds herself receiving social assistance, working as the superintendent in her apartment complex to help with the rent, and periodically taking in a boarder. Simultaneously, she experiences pain, fatigue, and depression. She said she was feeling trapped, but was somewhat relieved after Community Services paid for her medications. As a once-successful businesswoman, she now finds herself asking siblings and parents for assistance. She wants to work and be economically independent. She has now begun to understand the plight of the poor. "I've grown a great empathy for people who are on the streets," she told me.

ROBYN: I would like to earn enough money so that I'm independent again. I don't need to earn $100,000 a year. I need to earn enough money so that I can go get my supplements, so I can have a massage, so that I can pay my rent.

Michelle worked in a factory, but was unable to continue. She lived in subsidized housing and did not receive workers' compensation. While she had experienced asthmatic attacks earlier in life, she has since become sensitive to many foods and odours. (All the women in this book have developed some chemical and food sensitivities.)

MICHELLE: I started there when I was not quite twenty-three, and it wasn't long after that because of the solvents and the particles of rubber that float through the air that you don't even see. I didn't even recognize that they were there until I got a new fan, and within a day the blades of the fan were black ... and the rubber particles are extremely, extremely fine. It's like a very, very, very fine powder that they mix. And then, like the solvent, you're not supposed to get the solvent on your skin, and they gave us ... was it lamb's hide gloves to wear? But the solvent still got in your gloves, so ...

Not a person to complain, Michelle was laid off from work after a diagnosis of carpel tunnel syndrome, or—as her employers termed it—"repetitive motion." "[I] had a difficult time taking from anyone else or accepting help from others," says Michelle. "I always just feel that I'm taking advantage or ..." The part-time work she received from the post office did not supplement her income very much. To try to upgrade her education, she took several university courses but became ill again after a leak in one of the classrooms caused mould, forcing her to discontinue classes. The effort required to try for a disability pension was too much for Michelle and for most of the women in this study. They did not want to be seen as complainers or appear to be "taking from the system." This is contrary to the belief held by many that people with FMS are out to take advantage of employers or third-party payers and reinforces my view of the person who is conscientious to the extreme.

Full-time work/part-time work/forced retirement

Most of the women experienced a job loss or long-term disability or were forced to work part-time. This presents serious concerns not only because of the women's lost finances but also because they feel isolated and grieve for the work outside the home where there is more social interaction. Both political and social aspects are inherent in FMS, particularly with LTD claims, which are rampant with FMS diagnoses.

Sally speaks of not being able to work full-time. Although she complains of many environmental sensitivities, including an allergy to perfume that causes bronchial spasms, she does not ask for special favours at work. Sally says she is a very sensitive person; she does not want to burden others. She is fortunate to work in a scent-free environment where perfumes are not allowed. However, chemical odours are rampant in hospitals, and it is not known if they contribute to her sensitivities. It appears that, in spite of her distressing symptoms, she is not considering any kind of long-term disability. She enjoys her work, although there are some days when it is very difficult for her.

Vera speaks of stress in the workplace that finally forced her to take an early retirement. She recalls enjoying her work, but after twenty-five years in the same work environment, she was told by a new, younger manager that she wasn't doing her job properly. She was given a timeframe in which to come up with specific ways of improving her performance. However, this was an impossible task because she believed she was already doing a good job. This combined with other stresses in her life caused Vera to become more and more distraught. She did not miss time at work, even when it was very difficult to get up in the morning. She said her job as an office manager was very important, yet the pressures placed on her at age forty-eight were overwhelming. Vera, too, developed chemical sensitivities, not specifically from the workplace but from the environment in general. But more stress in her life caused hyperarousal of her nervous system and loss of self-esteem.

VERA: It was very degrading. And I talked to different people and it was—I talked to our human resource people—and it was funny because I got shifted into the human resources division. And, I mean, the director

was very nice, and she was a big, big help. And they sent me to a psychologist. They had me see a psychologist. Because I was very, I mean, I was
very emotional. I found it very hard to, you know, have all these people
know, you know, and, I mean, it was quite a let down.

It seems that the work environment precipitated extreme occupational
stress for many of the women, worsening their FMS symptoms. However,
like Michelle and Vera, many were expected to leave without compensation. If they did not leave work, they were either forced to take a leave of
absence, change jobs, or become part-time employees. It is probable that
highly sensitive women like those in this book could not physically or psychologically afford the hassles of long court battles. But how else could
these women prove that the workplace was not conducive to good health
and that their health had already been compromised? The symptoms of
FMS are invisible. More importantly, many do believe it is not an actual
disability or that the diagnosis itself is accurate. There are bitter arguments
about the reality of FMS as a disability and a real condition. The consequences of the workplace stressors on FMS symptoms, however, are very
real.

Disability Under Dispute

The American physician Hadler writes an impassioned plea to demystify
disability.[4] He identifies four categories:

- The disabled

- The disallowed

- The disaffected

- The disavowed

He critiques workers' compensation insurance in the United States. When
addressing compensation issues for those suffering muscular-skeletal
symptoms, he writes, "To qualify, one must be perceived to be so ill that
any employment is prohibitive." It is the same for those who suffer from

FMS or CFS. As invisible syndromes, the claimants do not visibly appear to be sick. They face the double dilemma of having to convince both the physicians and the third-party payers that they are ill. However, Hadler is not quite as comprehensive or as sympathetic as he may appear at first glance. In fact, he does not actually believe that FMS exists. In his controversial article "If You Have To Prove You Are Ill, You Can't Get Well," [5] he questions the diagnosis of FMS. If physicians are not united in their belief that FMS exists, how well are FMS sufferers likely to fare in the medico-legal domain?

The American physician Wolfe [6] has written the most vehemently against labelling FMS as a disability in spite of the fact that he was one of the originators of the modern-day concept and discourse about fibromyalgia. He maintains that while FMS is prevalent in all industrial countries, disability compensation is out of control. He writes, "As many as 25 percent of U.S. patients with FM have received some form of disability or injury compensation." He cites Israeli and Australian experiences in which work disability is not socially approved, and he uses these to argue that Americans "may be able to control the incipient FM epidemic as well." In his view, disability awards on the basis of FMS should be abolished. For those who are in chronic pain, he recommends a short, limited payment of one to two years. He believes that labelling FMS as a disability should cease, saying that the problems are psychosocial. I agree somewhat, although I would argue that the physical symptoms are real and significant. Why does labelling a syndrome as such mean support should not be given? Wolfe is against support groups such as those organized by the Arthritis Society (Canada) and Arthritis Foundation (U.S.); he believes they uselessly promote medicalization and actually prolong illness. Yet if he believes that the difficulties are psychosocial, then it would follow that support groups would provide comfort for sufferers as they share the enormous physical, economic, and social problems of FMS. While I agree that the *cause* of FMS is psychosocial in nature, I do not believe that it is psychosomatic. Rather, an over-stimulated nervous system creates a medical condition. In short, social structures medicalize FMS, or, in other words, FMS is socially constructed.

Wolfe's harsh position on FMS, which blames the victim, is one those of us with the syndrome find difficult to read. He does little to help solve the issues we are faced with in our daily struggles. This is ironic, given that Wolfe was primarily responsible for coining the condition in the 1970s along with other Canadian and American colleagues. Now his vocabulary is rampant with concepts of neurosis and failure.

How helpful has it really been to read his dogmatic position? I do agree that it is neurological at this point (that is, the nervous system is chronically over stimulated), but is it my fault that I have it? Was I responsible for the difficult life issues I have had to face? Is it a weakness of my personality? With physicians like him, how will we ever get to the badly needed solutions and answers? The cause is psychosocial in nature, and FMS people have become victims of societal dis-ease. Yet, I don't feel like a helpless victim. It's all very frustrating. But is it just FMS he is talking about, or are there other conditions like chronic fatigue, environmental illness, asthma, multiple chemical sensitivities, migraines, and allergies, to name a few, that he might also consider totally psychological in nature? Where could this end? Particularly when these conditions primarily affect women!

The Body/Mind Dis-Connection

The view that all knowledge can be verified by empirical science is called "positivism." Modern-day medicine is caught in the bind; unless there are physical causes for diseases that can be verified scientifically, they do not exist. Anecdotal data are generally not considered scientific. In this separation of mind and body, the body is treated and viewed as a machine that can catch pathogens, become physically challenged through noticeable injuries, or develop malfunctioning organs.

Consider this decision by a Canadian judge in Alberta[7], cited in the section "Physicians and the Law" in the *Ontario Medical Review*:

In a controversial decision, an Alberta judge has decided that fibromyalgia does not exist as a physical condition. Those who claim to suffer from fibromyalgia, the judge says, are hysterics who are unable to deal with the stresses of life, and who have converted that stress into acceptable physical symptoms.

We can only speculate about the difficult relationships among physicians who must diagnose, judges who must rule, and third-party payers who must compensate claimants. Conversely, there is this 1998 ruling[8], also from the province of Alberta:

> Edmonton—A ground-breaking decision by an Alberta court has allowed a woman with chronic fatigue syndrome to qualify for long-term disability benefits from the insurance company she worked for when she contracted the illness. The March decision in Edmonton Court of Queen's Bench is the first case in Canada to recognize chronic fatigue as an organic illness and not the product of a psychiatric disorder.

The medical view of FMS is conflicting. While there are many who choose to believe that there is a viral, genetic, or chemical cause yet to be found, there are others who believe FMS is a major psychological abnormality rather than an intuitive gift. It is believed by many to be either/or rather than multifactorial. Still others, with the interests of those who suffer at the heart of their views, sincerely believe that FMS is a bona fide illness or syndrome . The ways in which FMS as a syndrome is socially constructed is a political process with interplay between the various competing views of medicine, third-party payers, the legal system, and the people with FMS. Writing about the concerns regarding how women are often labelled as pathological, Schrager[9] points out that "the pathologization of women becomes a means of avoiding a larger social crisis in gender arrangements." Depression plays a big part in FMS and CFS; therefore, it is seen by those who believe that women are prone to hysteria that this hysteria is the primary cause of these conditions. That is, if "gender arrangements" are not taken into consideration, women become the target of blame for their own perceived inadequacies.

In her significant book *What Makes Women Sick*,[10] Lesley Doyal writes:

> On the one hand, "nervios" or "depression" can be seen as a complex physical and psychological response to the contradictory and demanding reality of so many women's daily lives.... In some instances they may be a culturally acceptable way of expressing anger and grief when no alternative outlets are permitted. It is also clear that a serious case of "nervios" is often a cry for help or a means of achieving change when the individual concerned is otherwise powerless.

It is HSP women (and some men and some children) who are prone to FMS, in my view. However, herein lies the paradox. On the one hand, I believe that there is a certain type of woman who is more likely to develop FMS, while on the other hand I do not wish to classify FMS as a psychological disorder. I do not accept the view that women with FMS are hysterical, out of control, or psychologically abnormal. Aron says that only the HSP knows the trait from inside. It is therefore necessary for a different paradigm to emerge, one which does not silence those who are afflicted.

Doyal further writes:

> It is clear that biomedicine has generated valuable knowledge that has been used to improve the health of individual women. But, as we have seen, this understanding is often partial and sometimes erroneous. This is because research has selectively ignored many of the biological differences between the sexes while paying little or no attention to the particularity of women's psychological and social circumstances.[11]

I confronted a dilemma as I read an article on FMS written in the *New Yorker*[12] that has caused quite a stir on the Internet among those who are genuinely, for personal reasons, interested in FMS. It is difficult when discussing FMS to sort out what is demeaning while preserving what is helpful. This article suggests that "fibromyalgia has recently become a matter of national concern." The author, Groopman, writes of the millions of dollars spent by the National Institutes of Health in the U.S. for research purposes. He writes, "The debate over diagnosis and treatment has become so heated that it has polarized medical specialists; choosing a doctor has become tantamount to adopting an ideological position."

A woman fictitiously known as Liz is quoted in the article saying that having FMS is like "being in prison in your body." She says she will not "see any doctor who questions the legitimacy of what I have." In this same article, Groopman frequently quotes Wolfe, who believes that the label of FMS is a convenient diagnosis for lawyers arguing for disability. Wolfe is cited as saying:

> If we underplay this [FMS], it will come down to a more minor label or disappear. We should diagnose it less. I think we should stop using the "F" word with patients, since it doesn't help them get better.

This article points out that there are six million Americans who have been *diagnosed* with FMS and that the majority are Caucasian. While Caucasian people may be diagnosed more often, they are certainly not the only ones to suffer from FMS. I believe that many who suffer from FMS do not trust the health-care system, do not visit doctors often, or perhaps cannot afford to see physicians in the first place. While it may be so that Caucasians make up the majority of people who are diagnosed, the real issue involved is in making oneself vulnerable to discussing a condition that is not legitimated by all health-care professionals, in particular those who are less privileged either because of race or economics. It is more likely that they do not acquire the FMS diagnosis. Many of the statements in this article could cause distress among many FMS sufferers. However, the article does make some important points, in particular, about the issue of the mind/body connection. The words of Dr. Bohr, a neurologist, suggest that he is of the body/mind ilk. Yet his language is one which is linked to a psychological disorder that implies mental illness of those with FMS.

Doyal,[13] a writer who discusses issues about the medical model of disease writes:

> Attempts to explain the causes of disease primarily by reference to specific biological hazards are too limited. They rarely explain the social and economic aspects of the environments within which such pathogens flourish ... Because the biomedical model focuses almost exclu-

sively on the material rather than the mental dimension of the "patient," it can offer little help in clarifying and explaining such experiences. In particular it is often of little use in understanding psychological distress and disability.

Depression, Psychiatry, and Mood-Altering Drugs for the Highly Sensitive Person

Most of the women in this book have taken medication for depression and/or had been to a psychiatrist or psychologist. Some found the experience of a psychiatrist helpful; others did not. In this same *New Yorker* article, Dr. Arthur Barsky, a psychiatrist at Harvard University, fails to understand that the people who are prone to FMS have a particular personality trait rather than a mental illness. Aron describes the HSP as one who has a "remarkable ability."[14] This gift is described by Aron:

> Most people walk into a room and perhaps notice the furniture, the people—that's about it. HSPs can be instantly aware, whether they wish to be or not, of the mood, the friendships and enmities, the freshness or staleness of the air, the personality of the one who arranged the flowers.

Should this intuitive, well-developed sensitivity be described as either a disability or a psychological abnormality? In my view, one with this ability (not *dis*ability) often becomes easily over-stimulated in a fast-paced world where demands and expectations are often overwhelming. Furthermore, being unable to tolerate so much mental and environmental stimulation can cause the nervous system to eventually become ultra-sensitive to smells, sounds, bright lights, and even people. As a body overreacts almost continuously to stimuli, the pain, fatigue, sleep disturbances, depression, and other symptoms become so chronically intense as to cause a physical "disability." It is only in that context that I am comfortable with the concept of disability as it applies to someone with FMS (or CFS). However, it is not a psychological "disorder," but rather an *ability* that Aron believes is inherent in 15–20 percent of the population and should be nurtured and cared for with compassion and respect. Aron writes that HSPs try to be like others, and being unable to do so leads to more over-arousal and distress. Even some animals are more sensitive than others.

We once had a dog named Jacob, a miniature poodle. This species is considered to be highly intelligent but very sensitive. He did not respond well to harshness; his personality was described as high strung. In fact, he was afraid of loud noises and turmoil in his environment and would easily become over-stimulated. Not a good environment for him in a household with three active young boys. We thought of sending him to a dog therapist.

BECKY: It just seems in my mind like a big swirl of events from that hysterectomy, right on to the next two years of just trying to find out what was wrong, nobody taking it very seriously, and me thinking, well, it's just me, and I'm lazy and, you know, I'm just dwelling on things that I should just put behind me now. And when I finally did go to my doctor and say, "Look, I don't know what's wrong, but I don't feel like me; in fact, I don't even know who me is right now," [I] broke down into tears, and he sent me to a psychiatrist.

JANE: I see a psychiatrist, and I have been seeing him for the last seven years approximately, because my doctor, that is my GP, he really doesn't seem to know a whole lot about fibromyalgia, and I don't really get the feeling that he's all that interested in learning.

BARBARA: Twenty-five years ago while under considerable stress, I went to see a psychiatrist who wanted me to go on an anti-anxiety medication. I had just been stalked for several months and then later was in a family situation with two teenage stepchildren and three teenage children of my own and a work situation that was stressful. The challenges were such that the medication did not help much, nor did meeting with her once a week to discuss my medication dosage. After three months, I ceased taking the medication and knew that this was not the path I needed to take. Fortunately for me at that time, I met with a psychologist at a local hospital who taught biofeedback and meditation techniques.

It is little wonder that mood-altering drugs do little for the highly sensitive person who is easily aroused and who can feel the nervous system overreacting to stimuli. It is not anxiety in the usual sense of the word, as the psychiatrist suggested to me. A good therapist can help the HSP to view her traits in a neutral or positive fashion without the encumbrance of a negative label, such as the kind of helpful work that is done in "freeze frame." This kind of instant therapy teaches the person to look inward in moments of stress and, with practice, control some of the effects of external stimuli.

Those of us with FMS, CFS, or EI are often labelled as psychologically inept. Consider this fragment of a demeaning letter from an administrator shared with me by a woman who had applied for disability because she was not able to work in a "sick" building. The language of this letter was very telling:

> EIS as a psychological or psychogenic disorder: Individuals who develop EIS are, generally, predisposed to the development of this type of illness, either through certain personality traits or early life experiences. These individuals lack appropriate coping mechanisms, and instead rely on psychological defences, to deal with day-to-day life experiences. In other words, these individuals lack the usual internal means of coping with external stressors posed by everyday life. This inherent absence of coping mechanisms constitutes the non-work-related component of EIS. The actual onset of EIS, however, is often triggered by the workplace, and again, the actual trigger or onset event(s) may vary. What is consistently found, however, is that the physical symptoms experienced by EIS sufferers are a physical manifestation of an underlying psychological disorder.

The Role of the Courts

Ultimately, whether a person is considered disabled, unable to work, and eligible for compensation will depend upon the court system. While the procedure differs from one country to another, the results of court decisions regarding insurance contracts appear to be somewhat arbitrary and often conflicting. Here are some brief Canadian examples:

1. In *Fulton vs. Manufacturers Life Insurance*[15] 1990, the Nova Scotia claimant was awarded disability after a disputed court case based upon the evidence provided by the family doctor. A rheumatologist stated that the claimant was disabled because of fibromyalgia and "poor coping techniques."

2. In *Martin vs. Mutual of Omaha*[16] 1991, an Ontario woman who worked in a production line as a labourer was awarded disability compensation for her FMS, but her rheumatologist said, "Again, I must stress that this is not because of physical limitations, but rather because of *perceived* pain."

3. In *Cook et al vs. Walkers Wharf Ltd. and Davis*[17] the plaintiff, a woman who was in a motor vehicle wreck, was awarded damages in 1992 because she had developed fibromyalgia after the accident.

It can be seen that in the first two examples the language refers to "inability to cope" with life situations and "perceived pain." This type of discourse minimizes the experiences of the sufferers and silences those who need to give voice to their stressful lives.

The Role of Attorneys and Physicians

The American attorney Scott Davis[18] has written extensively about disability benefits. He gives advice to those who wonder if they have a "good" disability case. He offers advice for those making a disability claim:
Step 1: You must believe that you have a valid disability case.

We've all heard the SSA disability horror stories ... but all too often I am surprised by the number of people who wonder whether they have a valid claim and it's worth their time to pursue it. In my opinion, over 80 percent of the individuals whose cases I review have a valid claim. If their claim is properly prepared they stand an excellent chance winning their case ... regardless of the diagnosis(es).

Step 2: Filing your application with SSA

You should file your application with SSA as soon as you meet any one of the following requirements:

- You have been out of work due to disability for twelve consecutive months

- It is *expected* that you will be out of work for a minimum of twelve consecutive months (if twelve months have not yet passed since you last worked)

- Your medical condition is *expected* to result in death

While FMS is not life threatening and does not meet the third criterion, nonetheless it can be seen that this particular attorney is describing many FMS sufferers with his first two criteria. In fact, he writes parenthetically: "yes, I am referring to the FMS/CFS crowd!"

Joshua W. Potter, Esq.[19] describes how important it is for patients to document their ailments and frequent visits to their doctors. (This is a common occurrence among those with FMS who go from physician to physician seeking a diagnosis). He writes that social security benefits are not easy to achieve with FMS, as proof of disability is difficult. However, according to Potter, the relationship between the attorney and the physician will help to make the physician's report more effective. It seems then that the person with FMS must make repeated visits to physician's offices, the physician must make detailed documentation, and the attorney must pull it all together to make an effective case for disability. Potter says that the medical report is key—that it is of "extreme importance"—to a successful disability claim. In short, it is up to the claimant to repeatedly visit the physician to build up a case for disability. Physicians in the U.S. must be familiar with the SSA "Listing of Impairments," Potter tells us. Then, of course, the patient will probably be examined by an SSA-approved doctor, generally after a long wait. It is usual for the request for compensation to first be denied, and this decision is then subject to an appeal heard by a judge. If the judge also denies the request (which is common), the person may appeal to the appeals council, and, after about seven months, its decision usually coincides with the judge. The long and convoluted process tires and frustrates the claimant who is already plagued with fatigue.

Kerry says that the insurance company paying for her long-term disability wanted her to return to work as quickly as possible in spite of the fact that she was the ninth person in her work site to be on long-term disability. It was found that the building was exacerbating her FMS, and she had developed EI. After being off work for a while, it was thought she could slowly return.

KERRY: So, on his [the rehabilitation counsellor] recommendation, I could go back to work, but I had to go through the work re-entry program. It would be like to go, say, half an hour for this week, an hour the next week, two or three times a week, like slowly introduce, get yourself back in slowly. Anyway, through my insurance company, like, they don't care, but for me it was, they don't care how sick you are as long as they can get you back so they don't have to pay for you. So that was his goal. His goal was to get me back to work. It didn't matter how I felt. Anyway, so he called me that they had a position for me at the X Building, which at the time I didn't realize was one of the sickest buildings that they could have put me in. So I went back to work in November, and I started having problems shortly after I got back. But I pushed myself, because I'm a person, like, I try to push as much as I can, which really is the wrong thing, because I made myself sicker.

Kerry was lucky. She was able to appeal and win her long-term disability case through the assistance of the physician in the Environmental Centre and her union representative. It was found that the room she was working in had mould, one of her allergens. Still, she expected they would bother her again, meaning the LTD was not secure or permanent.

Even more fortunate was Maddy, who for a short time was on 80 percent disability from the university insurance company. However, it was a long battle, and she eventually had to take an early retirement.

Jane explains, "[I was] working with my insurance company for the past probably year and a half, I guess. They were putting me through a rehabilitation program, you know, to try to get me to re-enter the workforce, although I don't know what they want me to do." Jane had enjoyed her career as a medical laboratory technologist but believed that the insurance company wanted her to re-enter the workforce as a secretary, which would have been a sedentary job for her and would cause more pain, and it was a job for which she was not qualified.

In 1980, the World Health Organization defined disability as a limitation of function that compromises the individual to perform within the appropriate range that is considered normal.[20] All of the women in this study would fit that definition.

Repetitive tasks—such as those involved in secretarial work, nursing, dental hygiene and many other so-called traditional women's jobs—generally cause more pain for the person with FMS. They cannot perform within a range considered normal. However, the aim of the third payer is to return the worker to any kind of work so that they no longer have to pay disability to the employee. The difficulty is that the person is often returned to a work environment that has no relationship to her own expertise or work history. This is just one more difficulty.

Is Trying for a Disability Pension Worth It?

The person with FMS is faced with serious economic concerns. Most of what is available for some relief is costly complementary medicine. In addition, bills must be paid, a cure is not possible[21] and permanent disability without compensation is very likely. However, the definition of disability remains vague in the case of the FMS sufferer. Most of us can walk, even if assisted by canes (unless there are other complicating conditions such as multiple sclerosis); generally we can use our arms and hands; and usually we are not bedridden every day, even though we may live with chronic pain and fatigue. However, we often have periods when the pain and fatigue are less problematic, and I am hesitant to have the reader perceive us as invalids. Even more significant is the fact that some of us are better off than others, particularly economically; there are no set criteria that can be generalized to all of us. There are degrees of FMS that vary from person to person and even within ourselves from day to day.

I still think of myself as a healthy person since I know this FMS will not kill me. On days when I am better, I feel optimistic; other times when I have an acute flare-up, I am despondent. But the very nature of this condition does not suggest we are not healthy, if we consider that our organs are fine and our bodies still "work!" I know though that I could not have fought a battle for any compensation. It would have exhausted me, and I wanted to continue to work. Those that do fight for compensation are the brave ones who have little choice left.

The decision to fight for compensation looms as one more assault on an already over-stimulated nervous system. However, what choices remain? Instead of viewing the person who looks for some form of monetary assistance as a malingerer, it is crucial that more respectful, less stressful, and better ways of applying for assistance are available to the person who can no longer work in environments that are not conducive to good health. The interviews with the women in this book lead me to believe that they all would prefer working outside the home in healthy working environments rather than staying home feeling isolated and abused by the system that perpetuates their condition. The solutions are not easy ones. They speak to broader social issues that have, to this point, been neglected in the discourse about fibromyalgia and chronic fatigue. They are political and economic problems that unfortunately affect women the most seriously.

The statistics are staggering in the article in the *Ottawa Sun*, dated Friday, October 16-21, 2005, in their special 5 part series (series on Chronic Pain). The author, Holly Lake, writes of estimates that there are more than one million people in Canada with fibromyalgia. The cost to the Canadian economy for chronic pain is about $10 billion per year (and in the U.S. $62 billion). While not all those who suffer from chronic pain <u>do not</u> have fibromyalgia, all who do have fibromyalgia <u>do</u> have chronic pain. From the FM-CFS Canada statistics cited in this lengthy article, it is noted that if all

1 million patients lost their jobs it would equal $6 billion in lost taxes. The problem therefore is not just an individual one but affects every corner of society.

In the next chapter, I will present advice intended to help others who find themselves in similar circumstances.

10

Words of Wisdom from Wise Women

The women who live with chronic physical syndromes are the experts of their own bodies. While living with FMS allows women to understand others who also have chronic ailments, everyone does not respond to the issues in the same way. Each of the women in this study knows her own body very well, and, of course, some of the women are more debilitated than others. Some experience a period of remission on occasion, while others are unable to continue with the activities of daily living as they had done before. Most importantly, all have different ways of dealing with the frustrations and challenges of FMS. However, for everyone, the management of FMS is like being on a roller coaster. Many women have tried one approach after another with some or limited success. Others have succumbed to the intense, disabling effects of their condition and are unable to do much more than survive.

Coping[1] is a common, contemporary word often applied to people with chronic conditions. It is a concept to which I do not respond well. Inherent in its meaning is the idea that one would dig in her heels, tighten her resolve, and make do with impossibilities—that is, adapt to the situation. With FMS, to cope means to make do versus being taken seriously and helped to find causes of the condition. It suggests that money for further research and treatment for those who suffer from FMS is not a high priority. Women have always coped with adversity, but I believe that most do more than that. The inverse of coping seems to be psychologically falling apart and not looking for answers to troubling questions about the condition. The women portrayed in this book are survivors, even in the face of uncertainty and the invisibility of their condition. Their words of wisdom are uplifting as they portray a deeper understanding of how they are learning to look after themselves following a lifetime of intuiting and looking after others. They are learning to take control of their own bodies, finding ways to be supported, and taking control of a difficult life situation. When asked to give advice for others, they looked back at their own responses to FMS and presented positive words of encouragement.

LOUISE: Don't feel guilty about being sick. Another thing, do try to enjoy yourself; Try to do things that make you happy. And you don't owe anybody anything, unless you feel like you've got to do this for this person. Mother has to be looked after, or whatever, you're, now it's your turn, you're sick and I don't mean to be totally selfish, but recognize that it's you. You have to look after you.

JANE: You know, you have to ... you have to find support where you can get it, wherever you can get it! And like I said earlier, you know, I don't know what I would do without my psychiatrist, I truly don't.

AMY: I have been very lucky. I was diagnosed in one shot. I didn't have to go spend ten years trying to figure out what the heck was wrong and be told I was crazy. So I was diagnosed in one shot, and I lucked out with a family physician who knew a lot about the condition and a rheumatologist who knew a lot about the condition, and they were saying, from day one almost, "You are going to have to find your own way with this condition. We can give you some supports and some things. We'll tell you things that we see work, but you are going to have to find your way." So I was given a lot of, not only given a lot of permission, but I was actively encouraged to find my way. And I was really sorry for people who, mostly women, who don't get that kind of message right up front and are somehow told, "You're helpless, and there's nothing you can do," or, "Here, I'm going to give you the answer." Because the answer changes from day to day. There's absolutely no way that anybody can help, really; you figure out what's going to work. And even I don't know what's going to work in different circumstances. You start out as a novice, and you try stuff, and it doesn't work, and you don't recognize patterns; you don't see them. Now I'm getting much better at recognizing what I think are subtle patterns, subtle interactions, and I'm getting better at thinking about how can I stop this now, how can I interrupt this now, allowing this to get too serious.

While there are variations among the women in terms of how each could take control of her own situation, it is dangerous to suggest that there is one specific answer to all of the difficulties encountered when living with FMS. The American Emily Martin[2] writes about how women's lives are shaped differently. She poses these questions:

> What are the main categories by which we in the United States think and act in the world?

> How do occupants of particular places in that world—such as women in different social and economic positions—see these categories?

> Can we speak of one homogenous view of the world, or do things appear very different if one looks with the eyes of a woman? A middle-class woman? A working-class woman? A black woman?

I did not find that race, age, or social class present different pictures of the symptoms. All of the women experience sleep disruptions, fatigue, pain, and periods of depression, albeit to varying degrees. The woman who is the most economically privileged of the group is more physically debilitated from all of those symptoms, in spite of trying various therapies for relief. It is true that those who are able to afford complementary therapies and who take advantage of that privilege are able to try different modalities. In spite of that, I do not see any long-term relief from FMS[3] for any of the women, though some seem to experience a degree of remission on occasion not related to a particular therapy. Some types of modalities are more effective than others, and finding what works seems like trial and error.

I have spent a great deal of time and money trying to find the best approach to my condition. I believe I have tried most of the different kinds of complementary treatments. I have found that water walking, body work, meditation, walking and "freeze frame" are the most effective for me. While yoga has helped somewhat, the practice has, on occasion, been less helpful than water walking, where stretching takes place underwater. I asked the women what advice they can give others who have fibromyalgia.

JANE: The advice I would give anybody is to find a doctor who is either aware of fibromyalgia or is willing to learn about it to better be a source of support to you. Find a good therapist [psychiatrist or counsellor].

LOUISE: Well, I would advise them to, first of all, find anything that works, that is not addictive, but something, a drug, that makes them sleep well. I think that to get a good sleep is very, very important. I figure half the battle is gone if you get that.

JEAN: Advice to someone who has fibro … learn as much as possible about the condition, and try as many of the techniques as possible to deal with the disease. Exercise, stretch, rest, try alternatives such as massage, electrotherapy, acupuncture, or whatever is possible. Keep moving as much as possible … at the same time being careful not to get overtired. Try to get help with establishing a better sleep schedule … possibly using Elavil. Avoid stress as much as possible. Learn to set priorities, and pace yourself. Proper nutrition will certainly help ease some of the symptoms.

Lisa Lorden, whose Web site I cherished but is no longer available, had valuable information about FMS and the holidays. It is now close to Christmas; I explore this season and what it does to people. Those who do not suffer from any kind of chronic condition find this month hectic. How about those of us with FMS? The decision to have a flu shot is one I grapple with every autumn. No one can tell me for certain if FMS/CFS people should have the vaccine. I get overtired from the holidays, and the stimulation is so bad for me. Then I develop a cold or flu. Lisa Lorden has helpful tips, mostly about recognizing how much we tend to push ourselves to try to continue the same traditions of the past. Next year, will I do the same? I don't seem to learn from past mistakes.

Diane has said that therapeutic touch has been very helpful, describing it as "amazing."

DIANE: The advice I would give others is to educate themselves … finding out what things have helped others whether it is exercise, an alternative solution, vitamin therapy … and most of all try to have a positive attitude even though sometimes it's so hard to have.

LESA: We should be more expressive ourselves [telling others how we feel] and not worry about, you know. We should try it out on our closest friend or our sibling or someone that we trust, try, try being honest. Because, really, it's a matter of being honest.

Mandy said that on gloomy days she has to be around people even if it means going to a mall. She said that it is important to do "an activity that will take you outside of your home or outside of your comfort zone and to transmit that into helping somebody else." Sally's advice is to "take time to smell the roses, one day at a time." From a more physical perspective, Vera said that exercise is a must for fibromyalgia, particularly walking. She also finds that her hot tub relaxes her muscles. I, too, have found that hot baths with Epsom salts are necessary for relaxation. Hydrotherapy, a technique of submersion of hot then cold water, has also been somewhat helpful for aching muscles. Most of the women in this book could not walk very far or could not walk every day. They found it difficult to feel positive about themselves when there were so many ups and downs and good days and bad days. Generally, most forms of exercise are relatively competitive, which is not a characteristic that those with FMS should strive for, even if the competition is with themselves. Walking for ten minutes one day may be all that can be done on that day, whereas a day of thirty minutes might seem like a victory. Leanne best sums this up in her advice to other women. "Note your successes in terms of *when* you're able to do things, to make a big thing of it." She speaks of being able to actually do two loads of laundry at once, which for her was an accomplishment.

It seems then that we all had great expectations of ourselves as high achievers who could take on many responsibilities for ourselves and others. But, as our energy waned, muscles stiffened and pain and fatigue set in, we all still wanted to be like we were before. However, being like we were before is why we have fibromyalgia. Being ultra-sensitive, curious, and intuitive means having a gift of anticipation about the feelings and needs of others, but it also means that we place increasing demands upon ourselves, by ourselves, to try to meet these self-inflicted responsibilities. It is only when this gift is used carelessly to the exclusion of our own health that it becomes a liability instead of a gift to be treasured.

Here it is now, my opus. The initial reason why I wanted to write this book has evolved in the writing. I learned so much about myself through this process, especially about how difficult it is to change patterns of behaviour. As I try now to stop the adrenaline high I get from stimulating events, I am aware of how highly addictive my behaviour has been. I want to fix things if I come in a room where everyone is not at ease. I want to take care of those I love to the exclusion of my own needs. I am overly conscientious; I push myself beyond my limits; and I am always "on duty." But I can work on letting go by reframing my responses to stimulation. I am not personally responsible for the pain of the world. I am so fortunate to have been able to learn more about myself through listening to these wonderful women and their courageous stories.

Writing about ill people as storytellers, Arthur W. Frank[4] notes, "One of our most difficult duties as human beings is to listen to the voices of those who suffer. The voices of the ill are easy to ignore, because these voices are often faltering in tone and mixed in message, particularly in their spoken form before some editor has rendered them fit for reading by the healthy. These voices bespeak conditions of embodiment that most of us would rather forget our own vulnerability to. Listening is hard, but it is also a fundamental moral act; to realize the best potential in postmodern times requires an ethic of listening." Frank calls people who suffer "the wounded storytellers." I hope that these wounded storytellers have provided voice to those who live daily with invisible suffering.

11

Women Revisited

While it was not possible to contact each of the women six years or even seven later, I was able to contact ten of them. Ten had moved, and I did not have access to their new addresses. I have included the ten women's updated stories and they reflect the life situation of most people living with the chronic condition for many years.

Jean

Jean's multiple sclerosis progressed in the intervening years, and she is now always in a wheelchair. She is able to transport herself from the bed to the chair and to walk enough to the bathroom from her bed.

She is still very active socially and spends a portion of the week as a volunteer teacher at her former school. She has become even more religious and is very active in her church. She remains high-spirited and, in spite of pain and fatigue, enjoys many activities such as visits with friends, piano playing, reading, cards, and Scrabble on line.

She needs more assistance in her activities of daily living and attends physiotherapy regularly. Jean continues to experience pain and other physical problems, but it is becoming more and more difficult to differentiate between the pain of fibromyalgia and multiple sclerosis. Her husband continues to be her caregiver.

Mandy

Mandy is no longer going to the pain clinic and says that her life is better now because her pain is under control. She is now on morphine permanently, which controls her pain and helps her to sleep well. The only time she feels worse is on a rainy or very cold day; then the pain in her arms, hips, and legs becomes very bad. While her injured arm, within which is a plate, is not as good as it should be, she says it is manageable. She still lives at home with her husband. She was not able to return to work.

Margot

Margot lives with her second-eldest daughter, who does all the housework, as she is still unable to do much for herself. She takes medication for nerve damage, pain, sleep, and depression. Her shoulders, hips, and elbows are in constant pain. She now finds walking up and down steps very difficult. She says that some days are manageable, but others are worse than previously. She is still somewhat isolated and unable to leave the home very much. She still misses social interaction and is unable to work either inside or outside the home.

Candace

Still working as a flight attendant, Candace now wears a back brace and experiences leg and shoulder pain. "I get by," she says. Some days she feels "out of it" because of fatigue. She is now better some of the time because of her medications.

She takes medications for severe arthritis. In addition, she is very keen on trazadone for sleep; it has been extremely beneficial, particularly when she has long overseas flights. She also takes Effexor for depression.

Chiropractor and massage treatments have helped her. One such helpful treatment is ART (active release technique) from her chiropractor, but it is painful, as she is almost unable to pull her arm backward. She does like water exercises, and often she does not have enough energy to do any exercises. Cold and hot weather are problematic, but now she is having hot flashes from menopause.

Sally

Sally says she does more for herself now and is somewhat better, although she is tired most of the time. She no longer works night shifts but is now working full time. She has regular massages, which help tremendously. She believes she is better than before and attributes this to the antidepressant, Flexeril. Her sleep patterns vary; some nights are better than others. Weather affects her greatly, particularly the cold.

Diane

Like Jean, Diane has multiple sclerosis, which has become more problematic than fibromyalgia. She had been going to a naturopath who had done acupuncture, but she found its effects to be short lasting. However, the naturopath moved, and Diane found it difficult to get to her new location. Currently, she is going to a chiropractor for treatment of muscle spasms in her spine, esophagus, and neck. She considers this to be the best thing she has done for a while. She says, "I didn't realize how much blocked energy I had in my spine and the problems that come from a spine out of alignment."

She had joined Curves for Women two years go but had to quit because the use of the upper-body-strength equipment caused burning down her spine.

Barbara

Since beginning this task of writing about our experiences, I have retired and spent a few years away from both the book and most of the women in this study. During that time, I traveled and enjoyed the time away from the hectic pressures of the workplace.

The first two years were relatively stress free. During that time, acute fibromyalgia attacks were scarce. Although I am always in chronic pain, the absence of acute attacks is a welcome relief (especially since I have lived with this demon since the age of twenty-five). During this time, I increased my walking to at least one hour per day and was feeling rather fit.

However, a foot injury, extreme cold weather, aging, and a crisis with my elderly parents (for whom I have major responsibilities) have precipitated acute attacks for the past few months. There is little doubt that caregiving is a big part of the psychic and physical pain I am currently experiencing. My nervous system is on high alert, and it takes a great deal of work to calm the over-stimulation. Massage therapy and chiropractic care are essential for me.

I cannot say if fibromyalgia intensity does or does not decrease with age as some have said. My hunch is that it is dependent upon life circumstances. Certainly without walking regularly either outside or in the pool, I do not feel as fit as I could. Hopefully, things will improve at least temporarily. Having had two years with a high degree of respite from acute attacks has given me some degree of optimism.

Michelle

Michelle recently experienced a traumatic, life-changing event. She has pains throughout her body, including aches in her knees, hands, and legs and in places where she never had pain before. She occasionally takes medication for pain but relies mainly on vitamins. She walks and can sometimes go to the gym, but she is careful not to overdo it.

She has not been able to return to work. She acknowledges that the recent trauma in her life and weather conditions have affected her, but she says she is "doing okay."

Maddy

Maddy has been able to control her pain with medications such as Gabapentin and extra-strength acetaminophen. She switched from OxyContin because she found Gabapentin to be more helpful. Pain must always be monitored and medications changed periodically from antidepressants to pain management.

Her life is very full with traveling, being a grandmother, gardening, and forms of exercise such as walking and cycling. Her leg tetany continues on and off. Drinking copious amounts of water helps the leg cramps somewhat.

Maddy is a very social person with many friends and a spouse with whom she travels. Her life is full regardless of the pain, fatigue, and chronic depression. Medications to keep the pain and depression under control allow her a better quality of life despite occasional breakthrough pain.

Becky

"Sometimes my fibromyalgia takes me by surprise," says Becky. She is usually in a state of "being careful" but "flying low." Becky still is on an antidepressant and uses Trazadone as a sleeping aid. She is working full time.

Intense weather changes are the most detrimental to her pain and fatigue. In particular, milder and wetter weather bother her the most. She is living at home with her grown daughter. Interestingly, her sister was diagnosed with fibromyalgia two years ago.

Not much has changed in terms of pain or fatigue except that she is now more careful about what she can and cannot do physically.

While I have not been able to reach all of the women, one of the pictures that does become clear from speaking with many of them is that pain control has become paramount in their lives, and newer medications have become available. For that reason, their lives are somewhat more manageable. In addition, medications in the form of anti-depressants have aided both depression and sleep challenges.

None of the women have said they are cured; rather, their lives are still filled with pain. However, they have become experts in living with chronic pain and fatigue. In other words, they are indeed at least coping. The women know more now than they did a few years ago in this era when massive amounts of information are available regarding medications. But the question remains: how do we manage our lives to the fullest while living with an invisible disability?

While my focus has been on women, I do not want to discount the pain of the hundreds of men and children who live with fibromyalgia—their stories are equally as valid. I believe them to be sensitive, caring, intelligent big and little people who are highly intuitive. Unfortunately, in a world fraught with one crisis after another, in a world where fear and terror are portrayed constantly to us in our everyday lives, it is likely that the number of sufferers will continue to swell. We can only hope that someday those who are highly sensitive will have the power to change a world that does not honour their gift.

Notes

INTRODUCTION

1. K. A. Wentz, C. Lindberg, and L. R. Hallberg,"Psychological function-ing in women with fibromyalgia: a grounded theory study," *Health Care for Women International* 25, no. 8 (September 2004): 702–729. In this study the authors uncovered a core concept that they called "unprotected self." They describe this concept as "mirroring childhood conditions and adult functioning." In other words, women were conditioned at an early age to behave in a certain way that did not allow for protection against being extremely helpful to others (hypomanic helpfulness) in adult life. It is this idea that reinforces the view of the ways in which women are psy-chologically programmed to become extremely vulnerable to the pain or needs of others.

2. B. Van Houdenhove, U. Egle, and P. Luyten, "The Role of Life Stress in Fibromyalgia," *Current Rheumatology Reports* 7 (2005): 365-370. The authors write of negative childhood experiences and life stress as con-tributing factors in fibromyalgia.

3. B. Van Houdenhove, "Fibromyalgia: A challenge for modern medi-cine," *Clinical Rheumatology* 22 (2003):1–5. This medical physician asks, "Should medicine only focus on symptoms and syndromes that have reached a full 'disease' status?"

CHAPTER 1

1. The descriptions of FMS symptoms are numerous, and can be found in many books on the subject. Among them are :

Leon Chaitow, *Fibromyalgia and Muscle Pain* (San Francisco: Thorson Publishers, 1995); Devin Starlanyl and Mary Ellen Copeland, *Fibromyal-*

gia & Chronic Myofascial Pain Syndrome (Oakland: New Harbinger Publications, 1996); Miryam Ehrlich Williamson, *Fibromyalgia: a Comprehensive Approach* (New York: Walker & Co., 1996); Devin Starlanyl, *The Fibromyalgia Advocate* (Oakland: New Harbinger Publications, 1998); S. C. Man et al., *Questions and Answers about Fibromyalgia* (Winnipeg, MB: Henderson Books, 1998). In the Web site www. fibrohugs.com there are 63 identified symptoms of FMS.

It is J. McSherry, "Fibromyalgia: Current Status," *Mature Medicine Canada*, (2000): 108, whose research I use here to point out that the most frequently used diagnostic test for FMS is applying pressure to certain *trigger* areas on the body, at which point the patient must then tell the diagnostician that the pressure is painful. While there are differences between trigger points and tender points (pointed out in the reference below from Wallace and Wallace), McSherry refers to these areas as 'trigger'. There are eighteen such paired points, and the patient must feel pain in at least eleven of them. The points of pressure for FMS are: (i) occiput, (ii) cervical, (iii) trapezius, (iv) supraspinatus, (v) second rib, (vi) lateral epicondyle, (vii) gluteal, (viii) greater trocanter and (ix) knees. Generally the pain is felt on both sides of the body which accounts for the eighteen points. Information about this diagnostic test can readily be found in most books on fibromyalgia. Some would argue that functional magnetic resonance imaging can be used to determine if a person has FMS, such as in R. H. Gracely, F. Petzke, J. M. Wolf and D. J. Clairw, "Functional magnetic resonance imaging evidence of augmented pain processing in fibromyalgia," *Arthritis Rheumatology* 46, no. 5 (May 2002): 1333-1343. However, the studies to date have been relatively small and inconclusive. While still others suggest that alogometer testing provides some evidence of FMS. However, currently, the most commonly used method for determination of FMS is still with trigger point pressure.

For an excellent historical review of this condition, suggesting that FMS has been around for a long time, read D. Wallace and J. Wallace, *Fibromyalgia: An Essential Guide for Patients and Their Families* (New York: Oxford University Press, 2003): chap.1.

2. Kerr's Web site is among many sites for those who are financially fortunate to be able to connect to the web. However, there are literally hundreds of web sites, and many of them are related to basic "what is it?" or "what can I do to cope" types of queries.

3. P. Palmer, "Pain and Possibilities,"*Feminism and Psychology* 6, no. 3 (1996): 457-462, discusses the "socioeconomic layers of pain." She refers to shame, fear, lowered self-confidence, and other losses because of social class issues. Many women in lower socioeconomic classes suffer in silence because of lack of confidence and the status differential between them and their doctors.

Add gender to this equation, and one can see from the work of E. B. Holmes and L. M. Purdy, *Feminist Perspectives in Medical Ethics* (Bloomington: Indiana University Press, 1992), that a feminist theory of pain reveals how oppression of disabled people adds to women's struggles with confronting their physicians. In addition read: Margo Maine, *Body Wars: Making Peace with Women's Bodies* (California: Gurze Books, 2000), 179. In the section titled "It's all in your head," she writes of physicians being twice as likely to discount women's health concerns as men's. In J. N. Clarke, "Chronic fatigue syndrome: gender differences in the search for legitimacy," *Australian and New Zealand Journal of Mental Health Nursing* 8, no. 4 (Dec. 1999):122, the author suggests that there is "a clear dichotomy between (a) the ways in which men and women experience the disease and (b) differences in the ways in which they are treated by the medical profession."

The illuminating book by Marni Jackson, *Pain: the Fifth Vital Sign* (Canada: Random House, 2002), does not specifically deal with women and pain but is a welcome addition to the literature on pain in general.

4. See K. M. Schaefer, "Struggling to maintain balance: A study of women living with fibromyalgia," *Journal of Advanced Nursing* 21, no. 11 (1995): 95-102. Also Chaitow, *Fibromyalgia and Muscle Pain*, p. 8, writes "86 percent females against 14 percent males" as the ratio of women to men who have FMS. Writing in the Winter 1993 *Ontario Fibromyalgia Association* newsletter, Thomas Romano, MD, from West Virginia says of FMS sufferers that the ratio of women to men is 10:1. Wallace and Wal-

lace (referenced above) write, "Even though one American out of fifty has fibromyalgia, the syndrome is distributed unevenly across the population, meaning 80-90 percent of patients with the condition are women", (p.8).

5. See *Arthroscope* (1998): p. 7, a publication of *The Arthritis Society*. However, there are many who dispute that fibromyalgia is indeed an arthritic condition. On page 1, Wallace and Wallace (referenced previously) state, "Fibromyalgia is *not* a form of arthritis, since it is not associated with joint inflammation."

6. Starlanyl and Copeland, *Fibromyalgia and Myofascial Pain Syndrome*, p. 7. The authors are not practicing physicians and, therefore, cannot give medical advice; however, their book is replete with information about current ways of "surviving" FMS, and their Web site is freely available to all at: http://www.sover.net/~devstar.

7. K. White and M. Harth, "The Fibromyalgia Problem," *Journal of Rheumatology* 25, no. 5 (May 1998): 1022.

8. F. Wolfe, K. Ross, J. Anderson, I. J. Russell and L. Herbert, "The prevalence and characteristics of fibromyalgia in the general population," *Arthritis Rheumatology* 38 (1995): 19-28. The reader can also find many other sources regarding FMS prevalence, with variability from 2–4 percent of the population as has been mentioned above in note 4.

9. Chaitow, *Fibromyalgia and Muscle Pain* (p. 8), says that between 3 and 6 million Americans are affected. Williamson, in *Fibromyalgia: A comprehensive approach*, says 2–4 percent of the population suffer from FMS. The statistics vary from one author to another and are speculative.

10. N. Hadler, "Fibromylalgia: La maladie est morte. Vive la maladie," *Journal of Rheumatology* 25 (1998): 1250-1252. This article has stirred up the current debate among doctors, especially rheumatologists, regarding FMS. Few can agree on its etiology and treatment, and whether or not it should be considered a disability.

11. For further information about this issue read: Starlanyl, *The Fibromyalgia Advocate*, p. 7, and Wallace and Wallace, cited in note 1.

12. See D. Starlanyl in M. Skelly and A. Helm, eds., *Alternative Treatments for Fibromyalgia & Chronic Fatigue Syndrome* (California: Hunter House Publishers, 1999): 22-27.

13. Majed Khraishi, "Evaluation of Fibromyalgia Syndrome," *Canadian Journal of CME* (February 2000): 111-119. This article brings up some very important points regarding evaluating FMS. The author cites a statistic that 17 percent of Gulf War veterans seen by rheumatologists reported FMS. However, it is difficult to know if the incidence is higher or lower among veterans given the recent publicity regarding Gulf War Syndrome, as it appears to be life threatening (while FMS is not considered so). Also included in the article is a useful chart of the trigger points that are used in the diagnosis of FMS.

Peter Radetsky, "The Gulf War Within," *Discovery* (August 1997): 69-75, asks why, if several hundred thousand American troops were in the Gulf, 'only' 110,000 have developed Gulf War Syndrome, and "Are some people more susceptible than others?"

Equally as controversial and puzzling is the debate regarding whether or not Chronic Fatigue Syndrome (CFS) is caused by a virus or chemicals. Jill McLaughlin, representing the National CFIDS Foundation in the U. S., presented testimony before the CFSCC on October 25, 2000. She strongly suspects that CFS is caused by a virus. While there have been numerous studies searching for a specific virus, none have been conclusive. I agree with Ms. McLaughlin that the traditional medical treatment of those with CFS has not been acceptable. More information on this testimony can be had by contacting amclaughlin1@mediaone.net.

14. Swedish research on FMS is prolific. Read S. Soderberg, B. Lundman and J. Norberg, "Struggling for dignity: the meaning of women's experiences of living with fibromyalgia," *Qualitative Health Research* 9, no. 5 (September 1999): 575-587.

15. J. G. Meisler, "Towards Optimal Health," *Journal of Women's Health* 8, no. 3 (1999): 313-320, writes about pain associated with aging and the areas of the body most commonly affected.

16. Years ago, Billie Jay Sahley, PhD, *Malic Acid and Magnesium for Fibromyalgia and Chronic Pain Syndrome* (Texas: Pain and Stress Publications, 1966), described a small study that showed malic acid and magnesium to be effective in the treatment of FMS (p.12).

17. C. A. Landis, M. J. Lenta, J. Rothermel, S. C. Riffle, D. Chapman, D. Buchwald and J. L. Shaver, "Decreased Nocturnal Levels of Prolactin and Growth Hormone in Women with Fibromyalgia," *J. Clin. Endocrinol. Metab.* 86, no. 4 (April 2001):1672-1678.

18. M. B. Yunus, M. A. Khan, K. K. Rawlings, J. R. Green, J. M. Olson and S. Shah, "Genetic linkage analysis of multicase families with fibromyalgia syndrome," *Journal of Rheumatology* 26, no. 2 (February 1999): 408-412.

19. J. C. Lowe, "Thyroid status of 38 fibromyalgia patients: implications for the etiology of fibromyalgia," *Clinical Bull. Myofascial Ther.* 2, no. 1 (1997): 47-64.

20. W. R. Neilson and H. Merskey, "Psychological aspects of fibromyalgia," *Curr. Pain Headache Rep.* 5, no. 4 (August 2001):330-337. Also: J. McBeth and A. J. Silman, "The role of psychiatric disorders in fibromyalgia," *Curr. Rheumatol. Rep.* 3, no. 2 (April 2001):157-164.

In W. Eich, M. Hartman, A. Muller and H. Fischer, "The role of psychological factors in fibromyalgia syndrome," *Scan. J. Rheumatol. Supp.* 113 (2000): 30-31, the authors write of expanding the view of regarding psychological factors to the biopsychosocial model in their article. These are but a few of the many articles linking fibromyalgia to psychology, thereby disputing the biology linkage.

21. Elaine Aron, *The Highly Sensitive Person* (New York: Broadway Books, 1996). It is the work of this author that has led me to the conclusion that it is the easily aroused nervous system of certain individuals (Aron suggests 15 to 20 percent of persons are HSPs) that eventually leads to FMS and CFS. She does not make the connection between FMS and HSP, but it is the combination of looking at HSP as she defines it, and reading that FMS is a dysfunction of the sympathetic nervous system, that has led me to this relationship.

Mark Pellerino, *Fibromyalgia: Managing the Pain* (Ohio: Anaheim Publishing, 1997), among others, has suggested that there is a predisposition to FMS that *may* be genetic. But I believe it is more likely psycho-socially induced in HSPs. While I believe that Aron's Self-Test regarding whether or not one is a HSP is not a very good indicator (as I believe that many women would respond in a similar way to the questions), her theory on sensitivity is well developed, and I therefore support her thesis about HSPs. Since FMS is primarily gender related and women generally are considered to be more sensitive psycho-socially, it does feel like a good fit. Another theorist who follows this line of thinking is Roger Easterbrooks. He uses the term *ultra-sensitive people* to describe such individuals, and like Aron, he believes they "pick up on most, if not all, of the subtleties that exist around" a person. He calls this being "deeply tuned in" on many levels whereby a person develops an "over-activated nervous system". For more information on his theory, visit the following Web site: http://www.ultra-sensitive.com/usp.htm.

Kerstin, Wentz, Lindberg, Lellemor and Hallberg, "Psychological Functioning in Women with Fibromyalgia: A Grounded Theory Study," *Health Care for Women International* 25, no. 8 (2004): 702-729, write of "compulsory sensitivity" described as hypomanic helpfulness that becomes self-regulating in adults.

In a highly technical article, D. J. Torpy, D. A. Papanicolaou, A. J. Lotsikas, R. L. Wilder, G. P. Chrousos and S. R. Pillemer, "Responses of the sympathetic nervous system and the hypothalamic-pituitary adrenal axis to interleukin-6: a pilot study in fibromyalgia," *Arthritis Rheumatology* 43, no. 4 (April 2000): 872-880, write that "FM(S) may represent a primary disorder of the stress system."

But it is to Dr. Jacob Teitelbaum from Maryland to whom I owe the greatest recognition. His experience and expertise with FMS and his newsletter "From Fatigued to Fantastic" have been extraordinarily helpful. In his Vol. 2, no. 1 (June 1998) issue, he writes on page 5 the following: "I find that I, and most patients with CFIDS/FMS, are 'mega-type A' overachievers. As a group, our *sensitivity and intuitive abilities are high* [my emphasis]. We had low self-esteem as children and tended to seek approval. This, combined with our *sensitivity to others' feelings* [my emphasis] caused us to avoid conflict and to try to meet other people's needs—at the expense of our own." He writes of our inability to say "no" and being unable to "defend our emotional boundaries." Furthermore, he contends that instead of resting when we encounter fatigue (from pushing ourselves to meet the needs of others), we push ourselves even further. I have checked this out with many of the participants in my study who say that this describes them perfectly.

22. See R. Wilkinson, "A Non-pharmacological approach to pain relief," *Professional Nurse* 11, no. 4 (1996): 222-224, and M. Hiscock, "Complex reactions requiring empathy and knowledge: Psychological aspects of acute pain," *Professional Nurse* 12, (1994):158-160.

23. R. Simms, "Fibromyalgia Syndrome: Current Concepts in Pathophysiology, Clinical Features, and Management," *Arthritis Care and Research* 9, no. 4 (1996): 315-328.

24. Karen Moore Schaefer, "Health patterns of women with fibromyalgia," *Journal of Advanced Nursing* 26, no. 3 (1997): 565-571. Also see K. Malterud, "Understanding women in pain. New pathways suggested by Umea researchers: qualitative research and feminist perspectives," *Scandinavian Journal of Primary Health Care* 16, no. 4 (Dec. 1998):195-198. Although this article does not discuss FMS specifically, it gives insight into the relationship between the attitude of medical professionals toward women's health concerns and the sense of trust that these women feel in the quality of their care.

25. K. Price and J. Cheek, "Exploring the nursing role in pain management from a post-structuralist perspective," *Journal of Advanced Nursing* 24 (1996): 890-898. Also, the late Patrick Wall was very influential in "the gate theory of pain." He, along with his colleague, Ronald Melzack, has presented theories regarding the neurophysiological basis of pain. Their book, P. Wall and R. Melzack, *The Challenge of Pain* (London: Penguin Science Books, 1996), is a classic that set the stage for further research in this area.

26. B. Hart and V. Grace, "Fatigue in Chronic Fatigue Syndrome: A Discourse Analysis of Women's Experiential Narratives," *Health Care for Women Intl.* 21, no. 3 (2000): 187-201.

27. J. A. Richman, J. Flaherty and K. M. Rospenda, "Chronic Fatigue Syndrome: Have flawed assumptions been derived from treatment—based studies?" *American Journal of Public Health* 84 (1994): 282-284.

28. D. S. Bell, *The Disease of a Thousand Names* (Lyndonville, NY: Pollard, 1991).

29. D. Buchwald in Skelly and Helm, op. cit.: 31.

30. Burton Goldberg, *Chronic Fatigue, Fibromyalgia and Environmental Illness* (Tiburon, CA: Future Medicine Publishers, 1998). This is an alternative medicine guide. See also Wallace and Wallace, referenced previously.

CHAPTER 3

1. Thomas Griner, *What's Really Wrong With You? A Revolutionary Look At How Muscles Affect Your Health* (New York: Avery Publishing Group, 1996). His view of muscle hypertonic spasm is related to a buildup of lactic acid. He writes (p. 53) that "lactic acid is produced when an animal cell metabolizes sugar anaerobically—without using oxygen". He says that the feedback *nerves* [my emphasis] are the only thing malfunctioning, not the muscles themselves. The buildup of lactic acid causes the pain, as the muscle is in spasm.

2. Pellegrino, op. cit., p. 19.

3. Another interesting read on pain in general is Dharma Singh Khalsa, *The Pain Cure* (New York: Time Warner Books, 1999). Also see Jackson, *The Fifth Vital Sign*, cited in ch. 1. It is a comprehensive book on pain that does mention fibromyalgia.

4. Moore Schaefer, op. cit. The women in her study spoke of the pain being worse when the weather was cool, rainy, or damp. The same holds true for me, the women in this study, and most of the women in this book.

5. Khalsa, op. cit., p. 19.

6. David Bell, *Curing Fatigue* (New York: Berkley, 1996), 139.

7. C. Henrikson, I. Gundmark, A. Bengtsson and A. Ek, "Living with Fibromyalgia Consequences for Everyday Life," *The Clinical Journal of Pain* 8, no. 2 (1992): 138-144.

8. G. Affleck, S. Urrows, H. Tennen, P. Higgins and M. Abeles, "Sequential daily relations of sleep, pain intensity, and attention to pain among women with fibromyalgia,"

Pain 68 (Dec. 1996): 363-368. Also, a classic read on pain is Elaine Scarry, *The Body in Pain* (Oxford: Oxford University Press, 1985). She writes of the difficulty to express physical pain, which is integral only to the person experiencing it. She says, "Whatever pain achieves, it achieves in part through its unsharability, and it ensures this unsharability through its resistance to language" (p.4).

9. J. Clarke, *Health, Illness and Medicine in Canada* (Oxford: Oxford University Press, 2000), 366-367.

10. A. Picard, "Depression assistance hard to get in old age," *The Globe and Mail*, January 9, 2002.

CHAPTER 4

1. Barbara Keddy, "Women Living with Fibromyalgia: The Body/Mind Connection," (paper presented at the Women's Health Conference in Victoria, British Columbia, April 29, 2000). This work deals with the psychic issues of shame and guilt as a result of living with a chronic condition.

2. A. Matsakis, *I Can't Get Over It: A Handbook For Trauma Survivors* (Oakland, CA: New Harbinger Publications, 1996). Especially significant is chapter 2, in which the author discusses the trauma to the central nervous system and the biochemistry of PTSD. Also in J. J. Sherman, D. C. Turk and A. Okifuji, *Clinical Journal of Pain* 16, no. 2 (June 2000): 127-134, we read that "PTSD-like symptoms are prevalent in FMS patients and may influence adaptation to this chronic disease [sic]." These authors from the University of Washington discuss symptoms of *arousal and hyper-vigilance* [my emphasis] which are congruent with my theory of the hyper-aroused nervous system.

Another article, Cynthia Chevins, "What Causes Fibromyalgia," Lycos Health with WebMD, http://webmd.lycos.com/content/dmk/ dmk,_article 5462092 (copyright 1996-2000), points out (p. 4) that "there is some evidence that PTSD actually results in changes in the brain, possibly from long-term overexposure to stress hormones." The article further states that "one study [not cited] has indicated that the incidence of sexual and physical abuse is higher in female patients with fibromyalgia than in the general population." I have no knowledge regarding any kind of sexual, physical, or emotional abuse of the women in my study, and I would not have violated their privacy to ask such questions. However, this article reinforces my view of the hyper-vigilant/hyper-sensitive/ultra-sensitive person.

3. Kaja Finkler, "A Theory of Life's Lesions: A Contribution to Solving the Mystery of Why Women Get Sick More Than Men," *Health Care for Women International* 21, no. 5 (2000): 433-455. See also Lesley Doyal, *What Makes Women Sick: Gender and the Political Economy of Health* (London: MacMillan Press Ltd., 1995) and Marian Pirie, "Women and the Role of Illness: Rethinking Feminist Theory," *Canadian Review of Sociology and Anthropology* 25, no. 4 (1988): 628-648.

4. Aron, op. cit., p. 8.

5. Elaine Aron, *The Highly Sensitive Person's Workbook* (New York: Citadel/Kensington Publishing Corp., 1999), 21.

6. In Chevins, op. cit., *hyper-vigilance* is described as an amplification of sensation in which people are *oversensitive to external stimulation* [my emphasis].

7. Jennifer Howard, "Gender Sensitive Health Planning—Why is it important?" *Canadian Women's Health Network* 3, no. 1 (Spring 2000).

CHAPTER 5

1. See especially Barbara Ehrenreich, *Complaints and Disorders: The Sexual Politics of Sickness* (New York: Old Westbury, 1973).

2. See P. Conrad, "Medicalization and Social Control," *Annual Reviews in Sociology* 18 (1980): 209-232.

CHAPTER 6

1. Simon Carette, "Management of Fibromyalgia," *Pain Research Management* 1, no. 1 (Spring 1996): 59. This doctor writes "the vast majority of patients with fibromyalgia report sleeping poorly and feeling unrested in

the morning. It is unclear whether this is due to a primary sleep defect or to the simple effect of chronic pain affecting the quality of sleep. Tricyclic agents such as low dose amitriptyline (10 to 25 mg. at bedtime) (18-20) and cyclobenzaprine (10 to 20 mg. at bedtime) (20, 21) have been shown in controlled trials to improve sleep and fatigue in one-third to one-half of the patients. This clinical benefit, when present, appears within the first two to four weeks of treatment. The drugs are somewhat less effective in reducing pain than in improving sleep, and their long term efficacy has yet to be demonstrated. For these reasons, these drugs remain of limited usefulness in the treatment of patients with fibromyalgia." Furthermore, these drugs can cause seizures in people with epilepsy.

2. Skelly and Helm, op. cit. Although this is one of the newer books on complementary therapies for FMS, there is no mention of an approach to better sleeping other than the usual medications prescribed by physicians.

3. Goldberg, op. cit., 312.

4. M. E. Williamson, op. cit., 12.

5. See D. Childre and H. Martin, *The HeartMath Solution* (San Francisco: Harper, 1999).

6. P. J. D'Adamo, *Eat Right 4 Your Type* (New York: G.P. Putnam's Sons, 1996). Many naturopaths are advocating this approach to better health. There can be little dispute about "we are what we eat"; foods obviously affect our health, yet I can find little that is written about avoiding foods that are not good for people with FMS. I am left wondering why so little has been written about this relationship.

7. K. M. Schaefer, op. cit.

8. Nanaimo News Bulletin, October 14, 2004.

9. See J. McGee, "Holistic Health and the Critique of Western Medicine," *Social Science and Medicine* 26, no. 8 (1988):775.

CHAPTER 7

1. Janine O'Leary Cobb, *Understanding Menopause* (Toronto: Key Porter Books, 1988).

2. See the newsletter *A Friend Indeed: for women in the prime of life* VII, no. 9 (February, 1991): 1-6.

3. Simone de Beauvoir, *The Second Sex*, translated by H.M. Parshley (New York: Knopf, Vintage Books, 1974): 301. Also see, S. de Beauvoir, *The Coming of Age*, translated by Patrick O'Brien (New York: Putnam, 1972). This is a classic on aging, and my all-time favourite.

4. In Elaine Anne Pasquali, "The Impact of Premature Menopause on Women's Experience of Self," *Journal of Holistic Nursing* 17, no. 4 (1999): 346-364, the author writes that "approximately 654,000 women [in the U.S.] have hysterectomies each year."

5. C. Mingo, J. Herman and M. A. Jasperse, "Women's Stories: Ethnic Variations in Women's Attitudes and Experiences of Menopause, Hysterectomy, and Hormone Replacement Therapy," *Journal of Women's Health and Gender-based Medicine* 9, no. 2 (2000): S27-S38. In this interesting study regarding ethnic differences and menopause, the authors state that the entire Navajo focus group asked "What's HRT?" (p. S32).

6. Sleep disorder is one of the many complaints of menopause. See L. Montero and I. Hernandez, "Social functioning as a significant factor in women's help-seeking behaviour during the climacteric period," *Social Psychiatry and Psychiatric Epidemiology* 28 (1993): 178-183. See also S. Welner, "Menopausal Issues," *Sexuality and Disability* 17, no. 3 (1999): 259-267. She writes on p. 261, "Insomnia has also been reported to be more frequent in menopausal women. The source of this sleep disturbance is unclear." Many others have written about the various symptoms of menopause and thousands of Web sites are available for perusal. However, the reader is cautioned that for the most part these symptoms are more common in North America and Europe, and that there is a scarcity of research about women in other countries. Furthermore, it is important not to view menopause as a disease. See P. MacWhannell, "Take the medical model out of menopause," *Nursing Times* 95, no. 41 (October 13, 1999): 45-46. She writes, "Drawing mainly on scientific discourses, medicine sees the menopause as an illness."

7. Poor concentration and memory loss are cited frequently in the menopause literature. The ways in which FMS sufferers describe it as

'brain fog' is similar to the words used often by the women who write to O'Leary Cobb's newsletter in the section called "The Exchange." In Karen Jensen, *Menopause: a Naturopathic Approach to the Transition Years* (Scarborough, Ontario: Prentice Hall Canada, 1999), the author writes that one of the symptoms of menopause is "memory problems and lapses, brain fog or 'weird' sensations in the head" (p.110).

8. The Web site http://www.fibromyhelp.com/qandas.html is a valuable source of information. Dr. Flechas writes: "Fibromyalgia appears to be most frequently present in women in a ratio of 20 women to 1 man. It is especially prevalent among those women in the age range of 35-55. The average age of first onset is 45." (accessed September 29, 2000).

Also, Carette, op. cit., writes "its prevalence in the general population increases with age, with values reported as high as seven percent between the ages of sixty and seventy-nine." It appears then that FMS in women occurs more frequently in the peri-menopausal, menopausal or postmenopausal years.

In J. Waxman and S. M. Zatzkis, "Fibromyalgia and menopause: Examination of the Relationship," *Post Graduate Medicine* 80, no. 4 (Sept.15):165-167, 170-171, a study of 100 women concluded that an estrogen deficit was the prominent factor in FMS. The majority of the study's participants had experienced menopause related to surgery. The average age of onset of FMS was forty-six. I do not concur with the authors that estrogen therapy should then be arbitrarily added to the treatment regime. Nonetheless, it is worthy of note that there is a possible relationship between menopause and FMS. However, this is only part of the picture, as children and men also experience FMS. This brings me back to my theory of the HSP who would have a tendency to develop FMS. It is likely that menopause is one more trigger that overstimulates the nervous system of the HSP and coincides with the development of FMS. Middle-age women are experiencing many more social and psychological stresses than ever before as they attempt to raise children, care for aging parents, work outside the home, and continue to be the primary household organizer.

9. S. Welner, "Menopausal Issues," *Sexuality and Disability* 17, no. 3 (1999): 259-267.

10. See B. J. McElmurry and D. S. Huddleston, "Self-Care and Menopause: Critical Review of Research," *Health Care for Women International* 12 (1991): 21.

11. P. Estok and R. O'Toole, "The Meanings of Menopause," *Health Care for Women International* 12 (1991): 32.

12. Janine O'Leary Cobb, "Reassuring the woman facing menopause: strategies and resources," *Patient Education and Counselling* 33 (1998): 287.

13. For a few cross-cultural studies on FMS see: D. Buskila and L. Neumann, "Assessing functional disability and health status of women with fibromyalgia: validation of a Hebrew version of the Fibromyalgia Impact Questionnaire," *Journal of Rheumatology* 23, no.5 (May 1996):903-906; J. E. Martinez, M. B. Ferraz, A. M. Fontana and E. Atra, "Psychological aspects of Brazilian women with fibromyalgia," *Journal of Psychosomatic Research* 39, no. 2 (February 1995): 167-74; C. Henriksson and C. Burckhardt, "Impact of fibromyalgia on everyday life: a study of women in the USA and Sweden," *Disability Rehabilitation* 18, no. 5 (May 1996): 241-248; L. Neumann and D. Buskila, "Ethnocultural and educational differences in Israeli women correlate with pain perception in fibromyalgia," *Journal of Rheumatology* 25, no. 7 (July 1998): 1369-1373; C. Lydell and O. L. Meyers, "The prevalence of fibromyalgia in a South African community," abstract, *Scandinavian Journal of Rheumatology* supp. 94, no. 8 (1992); E. Prescott, M. Kjoller, P. M. Bulow, B. Danneskiold-Samsoe and F. Kamper-Jorgensen, "Fibromyalgia in the adult Danish population: A Pravelence Study," *Scandinavian Journal of Rheumatology* 22 (1992): 233-237; M. Makela and M. Heliovaara, "Prevalence of fibromyalgia in the Finnish population," *British Medical Journal* 303 (1991): 216-219; and H. Raspe and C. H. Baumgartner, "The epidemiology of the fibromyalgia syndrome in a German town," abstract, *Scandinavian Journal of Rheumatology*, Supp 94, no. 8 (1992).

An interesting cross-ethnic study in the US involving African-Americans, Caucasians, Chinese-Americans, Japanese-Americans, and Hispanics regarding attitudes toward menopause and aging is that of B. Sommer, N. Avis, P. Meyer, M. Ory, T. Madden, M. Kagawa-Singer, C. Mouton, N. O'Neill Rasor and S. Adler, "Attitudes Toward Menopause and Aging Across Ethnic/Racial Groups," *Psychosomatic Medicine* 61 (1999): 868-875. Their literature review cites other cross-ethnic and cross-cultural studies of this nature as does the article C. Mercer, "Cross-cultural attitudes to the menopause and the ageing female," *Age and Ageing* 28 (1999):12-17. Another interesting study related to cultural and medical constructions of menopause is that of J. Winterich and D. Umberson, "How Women Experience Menopause: The Importance of Social Context," *Journal of Women and Aging* 11, no. 4 (1999): 57-73.

14. Germaine Greer, *The Change: Women, Aging and the Menopause* (Toronto: Random House, 1991), 250.

CHAPTER 8

1. J. Frueh, "Visible Difference: Women Artists and Aging," in *The Other Within Us: Feminist Explorations of Women and Aging*, ed. Marilyn Pearsall (Colorado: Westview Press, 1997), 214.

2. Aron, *The Highly Sensitive Person*.

3. Jacqueline Johnson Jackson, "The Plight of Older Black Women," in *The Other Within Us: Feminist Explorations of Women and Aging*, ed. Marilyn Pearsall, op. cit., 37-42. The author states, "What I believe is becoming a dangerous trend is the increasing pulls upon older Black women to belong to a multiplicity of organizations devoted to blacks, to women, to the elderly, and so on" (p.41). I have found little, however, that documents this intense caring for others is harmful to their health. Also see Karla F.C. Holloway and Stephanie Demetrakopooulos, "Remembering Our Foremothers, Older Black Women, Politics of Age, Politics of Survival as Embodied in the Novels of Toni Morrison," in *The Other Within Us: Feminist Explorations of Women and Aging*, ed. Marilyn Pearsall, op. cit., 177-195. While praising older women, these authors do not write of the burden this places on them: "My grandmother went through menopause in her mid-twenties. Her early menopause was significant in the

construction of our family. For us, it meant that grandmother extended her nurturing to several other children, related and not related" (p. 183). The Black woman as nurturer is easily found in the literature, but little can be found that speaks to the cost on the woman's emotional and physical health. Black women are caught among various myths and stereotypes such as "strong black women," "mammy," and "matriarch."

4. Childre and Martin, op. cit., p. 20, write: "It's critical to learn the difference between care and *overcare* [my emphasis]. Caring for yourself and others is an essential ingredient for a rewarding life. Unfortunately, caring can also be stressful. When our care goes too far, we experience what we call "overcare," a term that denotes a burdensome sense of responsibility accompanied by worry, anxiety, or insecurity. A host of problems result when we allow our care to become draining, including lowered immune response, imbalanced hormone levels, and poor decision-making." I believe that *overcaring* is related to intuitive understanding and anticipation of the needs of others and a resistance toward separating one's own needs from that of others.

5. L. Gordon, *Heroes of Their Own Lives* (New York: Viking, 1988).

6. Aron, *The Highly Sensitive Person*, 109.

7. J. Aronson, "Dutiful Daughters and Undemanding Mothers: Constraining Images of Giving and Receiving Care in Middle and Later Life," in *Women's Caring Feminist Perspectives on Social Welfare*, ed. Carol Baines, Patricia Evans and Sheila Neysmith (Toronto: McClelland and Stewart), 160.

CHAPTER 9

1. Read Chip Davis at cdavis@webtk.com. It is here on the Internet that I first heard of the mayor's proclamation.

2. G. McCain, R. Cameron and J. Kennedy, "The Problem of Long-term Disability Payments and Litigation in Primary Fibromyalgia: The Canadian Perspective," *Journal of Rheumatology* 16, Supp. 19 (1989): 174.

3. P. Moss, "Negotiating Spaces in Home Environments: Older Women Living with Arthritis," *Social Science Medicine* 45, no.1 (1997): 25.

4. N. Hadler, "The Disabled, the Disallowed, the Disaffected and the Disavowed," *JOEM* 38, no. 3 (March 1996): 248.

5. N. Hadler, "If you have to prove you are ill, you can't get well," *Spine* 2 (1996): 2397-2400.

6. F. Wolfe, "The fibromyalgia Problem," *The Journal of Rheumatology* 24, no. 7 (1997): 1247-1249. While the author cites the Australian and Israeli experiences, the Norway situation resembles the North American experience. In D. Bruusgard, A. Evensen and T. Bjerkedal, "Fibromyalgia—a new cause for disability pension," *Scandinavian Journal of Social Medicine* 21, no. 2 (1993):116-119, the authors point out that while fibromyalgia is a condition under dispute, "In 1988, fibromyalgia was by far the most frequent single diagnosis as a reason for disability pensions in Norway", p.116.

7. J. Sack and V. Payne, "Alberta Judge Denies Existence of Fibromyalgia," *Ontario Medical Review* (February 1995): 67. The authors cite Mackie vs. Wolfe, unreported, June 10, 1994 (Alberta Court of Queen's Bench).

8. R. Henderson, "Chronic fatigue syndrome an illness, court rules" (1998), http://www.edmontonjournal.com/news/alberta/042298ab2.html.

9. C. Schrager, "Questioning the Promise of Self-Help: A Reading of Women Who Love Too Much," *Feminist Studies* 19 (Spring 1993): 187. Although the author is writing about violence, not FMS, her quote is appropriate for my point.

10. Lesley Doyal, *What Makes Women Sick: Gender and the Political Economy of Health* (New Jersey: Rutgers University Press, 1995), 45. This is a very interesting read and one that has much applicability to the arguments I make.

11. Doyal, op. cit., 18.

12. J. Groopman, "Hurting All Over," *The New Yorker*, November 13, 2000, 78-92.

13. Doyal, op. cit., 16.

14. Aron, *The Highly Sensitive Person*, 4-5.

15. [1990] I.L.R.1-2620, as cited in John Verrier Jones and Diana Ginn, "Fibromyalgia: The Canadian Courts Have Spoken," *Journal of Canadian Rheumatology Association* (date unknown).

16. [1992] I.L.R. 1-2795, ibid.

17. [1992] 117N.S.R. (2d) 361, ibid.

18. Lisa Lorden, "Obtaining Social Security Disability: How to Begin the Process," http://chronicfatigue.about.com/health/chronicfatigue/library/uc/uc_sdavisbegin.html (2000).

19. Joshua Potter, "Physician Input Strengthens Claim: Helping Fibromyalgia Patients Obtain Social Security Benefits," *Journal of Musculoskeletal Medicine* 9, no. 9 (1992): 65-74.

20. World Health Organization: "The international classification of impairments, disabilities, and handicaps," World Health Organization, 1980.

21. At the same time that the *New Yorker* came out with its article on FMS, another journal did as well. In Alicia Sirkin, "Fibromyalgia falls to flowers," *Alternative Medicine*, 39, (January 2001): 76-85, a claim is made that Bach Flower Essences can sometimes be a cure for FMS. It is interesting to note, however, that not only did one of the Registered Bach Foundation Practitioners prescribe the flower essences, but she also took on the role of therapist. The woman described in the article fits the role of the HSP! It would seem that without therapy any kind of complementary medicine would be less than adequate.

CHAPTER 10

1. Dennis Turk, "Psychological Aspects of Chronic Pain," in *Alternative Treatments for Fibromyalgia & Chronic Fatigue Syndrome*, ed. Skelly and Helm, 205-208. On page 207 he describes three types of FMS "patients": The first he says are "dysfunctional"; they are said to have little control over their lives. The second group is referred to as "interpersonally distressed"; that is, they are thought to feel that they receive little support

from others. The third category he calls "adaptive copers." I believe that this kind of stereotyping is a demeaning and dangerous practice. I see little value in labelling people who may shift from one characteristic to another, or not even fit any of these categories. It is a structural-functional mode of describing people that suggests there is little mobility between the classifications. But more importantly, this kind of categorizing is not particularly useful because of its inherent gender, class, and race biases.

2. E. Martin, *The Woman in the Body: Cultural Analysis of Reproduction* (Boston: Beacon Press, 1987), 15. While the author specifically speaks of issues around reproduction, her writings have become classics among academics interested in issues of women and health.

3. Carol Landis, "Sleep Dysfunction and Fibromyalgia," in *Alternative Treatments for Fibromyalgia & Chronic Fatigue Syndrome*, ed. Skelly and Helm, 211.

4. Arthur W. Frank, *The Wounded Storyteller: Body, Illness and Ethics* (Chicago and London: University of Chicago Press, 1995), 25.

Fibromyalgia Resource List

ORGANIZATIONS

Arthritis Foundation
PO Box 19000
Atlanta, GA 30326
Arthritis Information Fibromyalgia (booklet)
1-800-283-7800
(Request information at no cost)

The Arthritis Foundation
Southern Maryland Chapter
(Check with your local branch)
1-410-544-5433
(Annapolis Fibromyalgia Support Group meets the third Monday of every month)

National Chronic Pain Outreach Association
7979 Old Georgetown Road, #100
Bethesda, MD 20814-2429
1-301-652-4928
(Quarterly newsletter on chronic pain)

The National Arthritis, Muscoskeletal, and Skin Diseases
Information Clearinghouse
9000 Rockville Rike
Box AMS
Bethesda, MD 20892
1-301-495-4484

Fibromyalgia Assoc. of Greater Washington (FMAGW)
13203 Valley Drive
Woodbridge, VA 22191-1531
1-703-790-2324
Fax: 1-703-494-4103
E-mail: mail@fmagw.org
http://www.fmagw.org
Quarterly newsletter: *Fibromyalgia Frontiers*, a source of the latest information on FMS and research
Monthly meetings with guest speakers
Membership: $25/yr. ($12/yr. students)

Fibromyalgia Association of Florida, Inc.
PO Box 14848
Gainesville, FL 3260-4848
1-904-373-6865

Fibromyalgia Alliance of America, Inc. (FMAA)
PO Box 21990
Columbus, Ohio 43221-0990
1-614-457-4222
Fax: 1-614-457-2729
Quarterly newsletter, source of latest information on FMS and FMS research
Support and membership
The Fibromyalgia Syndrome ($4.00 for this booklet)

National Chronic Fatigue Syndrome & Fibromyalgia Assoc.
PO Box 18426
Kansas City, MO 64133
1-816-313-2000 (24-hour information line)

Fibromyalgia Network
PO Box 31750
Tucson, AZ 85751-1750
1-520-290-5508 or 1-800-853-2929
Fax: 1-520-290-5550
http://fmnetnews.com
Newsletter (Fibromyalgia Network), educational materials

Seattle Fibromyalgia Association
PO Box 77373
Seattle, WA 98177
1-205-362-2310
Educational materials.

Fibromyalgia Association of Texas, Inc
5650 Forest Lane
Dallas, TX 75230

CAN (Activist group for CFIDS and FM)
PO Box 345
Larchmont, NY 10538

M.E./Chronic Fatigue Syndrome Society of Queensland Inc.
134 St. Paul's Terrace, Spring Hill
PO Box 938
Fortitude Valley QLD 4006
(07)3832 9322 or 1-800-000-376
Fax: (07)3832 9755
http://www.mecfsqld.org.au

Fibromyalgia Association of Saskatchewan
PO Box 7525
Saskatoon, Saskatchewan S7K 4L4
306-574-4711
Newsletter: *FM Bulletin*

Fibromyalgia Support Group of Winnipeg, Inc.
825 Sherbrooke Street
Winnipeg, Manitoba R3A 1M5
204-772-6979
Newsletter: *FMS Today*

Ontario Fibromyalgia Association
393 University Ave.
Suite 1700
Toronto, Ontario B5G 1E6
416-979-7228
Fax: 416-979-8366

NEWSLETTERS

Fibromyalgia Network
PO Box 31750
Tucson, AZ 85751-1750
1-800-853-2929
(Four issues per year)

FM Forum
FM Association of B.C.
PO Box 15455
Vancouver, BC V6B 5B2
(Associated with The Arthritis Society—BC Division. Four issues per year)

OFA Tender Points
Ontario Fibromyalgia Association
250 Bloor Street East, Suite 901
Toronto, Ontario M4W 3P2
(Associated with The Arthritis Society—Ontario Division. Three issues per year)

The Fibromyalgia Times
Fibromyalgia Association of America
PO Box 21990
Columbus, Ohio 43221-0990
(Four issues per year)

Fibromyalgia Frontiers
FM Association of Greater Washington
PO Box 2373
Centreville, VA 22020
(Four issues per year)

The Messenger
M.E. Canada
400 Queen Street
Ottawa, Ontario K1P 5E4
(Twelve issues per year)

National ME/FM Action Network
3836 Carling Avenue
Nepean, Ontario K2K 2Y6
613-829-6667

WEB PAGES

Fibromalgia & Chronic Fatigue
http://www.Fmnetnews.com/

Fibromyalgia Association
http://www.w2.com/Fibro1.html

Fibromyalgia & Chronic Myofascial Pain Syndrome
http://www.sover.net/~devstar

Exercise program for fibromyalgia
http://Familydoctor.org/handouts/061.html

http://www.hsc.missouri.edu/~Fibro/

Treatment of Fibromyalgia Syndrome
http://www.Futureone.com/~hunter/treat.htm

What is Fibromyalgia Syndrome?
http://www.fibrom-1.org/fibro.htm

Fibromyalgia Page
http://www.americanwholehealth.com/library/fibromyalia

Living with FMS
http://www.tidalweb.com/fms?
http://www.mbnet.mb.ca/crm/health/asmp/html

Arthritis Canada
http://www.arthritis.ca

Fibromyalgia.ca
Bedford Fibromyalgia Support Group
http://www.bedford.net/jelliser/index12x.html

Fibromyalgia Resource Centre
HealingWell.com

Fibro Friends Network
http://www.fibrofriendsnetwork.com

Consumer Wellness: Fibromyalgia
http://www.consumerwellness.com/fibromyalgia.html

Fibromyalgia information
http://www.ncf.ca/fibromyalgia

Fibromyalgia Network
http://www.fmnetnews.com

Fibromyalgia Patient Support Center
http://www.fmpsc.org/info/info.htm

ME/FM National Action Network (includes disability pension info)
http://www3.sympatico.ca/me-fm.action

National Fibromyalgia Awareness Campaign
members.xoom.com/nfac/home/htm

Therapy in Motion—Massage therapy
http://www.ncf.ca/massagetherapy

Fibromyalgia Resources
http://dwp.bigplanet.com/john1 123/fibromyalgia/

Fibromyalgia: Resources for Families
http://www.1clark.edy/~sherrons/topic_concept.htm

Chronic Fatigue Syndrome/Fibromyalgia
http://chronicfatigue.about.com/health/chronicfatigue/cs/fibromyalgia

Fibromyalgia and Chronic Myofascial Pain Syndrome (FMS/MPS) from
Dr. Devin Starlanyl
http://www.sover.net/~devstar/
found in: Health > Conditions and Diseases > F > Fibromyalgia > Clinical
Theory

Fibromyalgia Network
http://www.fmnetnews.com/
found in: Health > Conditions and Diseases > F > Fibromyalgia > Organizations

Fibromyalgia Association of Greater Washington
http://www.fmagw.org/
found in: Health > Conditions and Diseases > F > Fibromyalgia > Organizations

Arthritis Insight-Fibromyalgia
http://www.arthiritisinsight.com/medical/diseases/fms.html
found in: Health > Conditions and Diseases > F > Fibromyalgia

Gossamer's CFIDS/FMS Site
http://www.tertius.net.au/foothold
found in: Health > Conditions and Diseases > C > Chronic Fatigue Syndrome

FM/CFS/CFIDS/ME and more!
http://www.the-mac-lady.com/Fm_CFS_CFIDS_PR.html
found in: Health > Conditions and Diseases > F > Fibromyalgia

CFIDS CFS FMS M.E. GWS Directory
http://www.theriver.com/Public/cfids
found in: Health > Conditions and Diseases > C > Chronic Fatigue Syndrome

Colorado Health Net Fibromyalgia Center
http://www.coloradohealthnet.org/site/idx_fibro.html
found in: Health > Conditions and Diseases > F > Fibromyalgia

Info on CFIDS, FMS, NMH, POTS, MCS and related illnesses
http://www.homestead.com/CFIDS/infoplace.html
found in: Health > Conditions and Diseases > C > Chronic Fatigue Syndrome

Fibromyalgia Syndrome—Articles by Devin Starlanyl, MD
http://www.clark.net/pub/tbear/fms/fms-star.htm
found in: Health > Conditions and Diseases > F > Fibromyalgia > Clinical Theory and Practice

North American Chronic Pain Association of Canada
http://www.chronicpaincanada.org

The National Fibromyalgia Research Association
http://www.teleport.com/~nfra/

From Fibro North
http://www.fibronorth.com/links.html

Fibromyalgia Self-help group Online (Newfoundland and Labrador)
http://www3.nf.sympatico.ca/jmld

Better Life Now Inc. Relief for Fibromyalgia and Chronic Fatigue Syndrome Newsletter
http://www.cadvision.com/jonesd/News-Letter.htm

WILL SEND A PACKET ON STARTING A SUPPORT GROUP

Mary Anne Saathoff
Fibromyalgia Alliance of America, Inc. (FMAA)
PO Box 21990
Columbus, Ohio 43221-0990
Phone: 1-614-457-4222
Fax: 1-614-457-2729
(Also can order her booklet on FM for $4.00)

Kristin Thorson
FM Network News
PO Box 31750
Tucson, AZ 85751-1750
1-520-290-5508
http://fmnetnews.com
Subscription rate is $19.00/yr.
Canadian Residents $21 U.S. funds money order
Outside North America: $25 U.S. funds
Free information pamphlet

Joan Wackerly
The Florida Fibro News
PO Box 1484
Gainesville, FL 32604-4848
1-904-373-6865
(Subscription rate is $15.00/yr USA)
Free information pamphlet

Karen Samuelson
FM Association of Texas, Inc.
5650 Forest Lane
Dallas, Texas 75320

KOFF, Inc. (Kansas Outreach)
Rebecca Robbins
1216 Appleton
Parsons, KA 67357
1-316-421-3881

ONLINE SUPPORT

Fibrom-L (Fibromyalgia listserv)
To subscribe to Fibrom-L, send a message to: listserv@mitvma.mit.edu
Leave the message line blank. In the body of the message, write "subscribe
FIBROM-L." You will receive a confirmation and instructions to follow in
order to post to the list, unsubscribe, or change your options.

FMS-Chat (Support listserv)
Send all requests to: listserv@mitvma.mit.edu
Always leave the subject line blank. In the body of the message, write "subscribe FMS-Chat." You will receive a confirmation and instructions to follow in order to post to the list, unsubscribe, or change your options.

http://www.ncf.ca/fibromyalgia/sg_info.htm

VIDEOS AND TAPES

Fibromyalgia: Face to Face, a video produced by the Ontario FM Association is available for $19.95. To order, send a cheque or money order to the
address for the Ontario FM Association above.

Fibromyalgia and You (90 minutes) covers what FM is, including diagnosis and possible causes, approaches to treatment, and how to live with FM. To order, send a money order for $34.95 U.S. dollars to:
Fibromyalgia Information Resources
PO Box 690402
San Antonio, Texas 78269

Fibromyalgia Exercise Video, an exercise video designed for persons with FM, is available on loan from The Arthritis Society—Nova Scotia Division. You may borrow it by calling 429-7025 or 1-800-321-1433. You can also buy one by sending a cheque or money order for $24.50 payable to: OTMH Charitable Corporation Exercise Video. Mail to:
Oakville Trafalgar Memorial Hospital
Attn: Physiotherapy Dept.
327 Reynolds Street
Oakville, ON L6J 3L7

Fibromyalgia Stretch Video gives you thirty minutes of stretching exercises. Some proceeds from the sale of this video will go to FM research. To order, send a money order for $24.95 U.S. dollars to:
Fibromyalgia Stretch Video
PO Box 500
Salem, Oregon 97308

Bibliography

A Friend Indeed: for women in the prime of life 7, no. 9 (February, 1991): 1-6.

Affleck, G., S. Urrows, H. Tennen, P. Higgins and M. Abeles. "Sequential daily relations of sleep, pain intensity, and attention to pain among women with fibromyalgia." *Pain* 68 (Dec. 1996): 363-368.

Aron, Elaine. *The Highly Sensitive Person.* New York: Broadway Books, 1996.

Aron, Elaine. *The Highly Sensitive Person's Workbook.* New York: Citadel/Kensington Publishing Corp., 1999.

Aronson, L. "Dutiful Daughters and Undemanding Mothers: Constraining Images of Giving and Receiving Care in Middle and Later Life." In *Women's Caring Feminist Perspectives on Social Welfare*, edited by Carol Baines, Patricia Evans and Sheila Neysmith, 138-168. Toronto: McClelland and Stewart, 1991.

Arthroscope. The Arthritis Society, 1998.

Bell, David and Stef Donev. *Curing Fatigue.* New York: Berkley, 1996.

Bell, D. S. *The Disease of a Thousand Names.* Lyndonville, NY: Pollard, 1991.

Bruusgard, D., A. Evensen and T. Bjerkedal. "Fibromyalgia—a new cause for disability pension." *Scandinavian Journal of Social Medicine* 21, no. 2 (1993):116-119.

Buchwald, Debra. "Formal Diagnosis and Treatment of Chronic Fatigue Syndrome." In *Alternative Treatments for Fibromyalgia & Chronic Fatigue Syndrome*, edited by Mari Skelly and Andrea Helm, 30-34. California: Hunter House Publishers, 1999.

Buskila, D. and L. Neumann. "Assessing functional disability and health status of women with fibromyalgia: validation of a Hebrew version of the Fibromyalgia Impact Questionnaire." *Journal of Rheumatology* 23, no.5 (May 1996): 903-906.

Carette, Simon. "Management of Fibromyalgia." *Pain Research Management* 1, no. 1 (Spring 1996): 58-60.

Chaitow, Leon. *Fibromyalgia and Muscle Pain*. San Francisco: Thorson Publishers, 1995.

Childre, D. and H. Martin. *The HeartMath Solution*. San Francisco: Harper, 1999.

Clarke, J. *Health, Illness and Medicine in Canada*. Oxford: Oxford University Press, 2000.

Clarke, J. N. "Chronic fatigue syndrome: gender differences in the search for legitimacy." *Australian and New Zealand Journal of Mental Health Nursing* 8, no. 4 (Dec. 1999):123-133.

Conrad, P. "Medicalization and Social Control." *Annual Reviews in Sociology* 18 (1980): 209-232.

D'Adamo, P. J. *Eat Right 4 Your Type*. New York: G.P. Putnam's Sons, 1996.

de Beauvoir, Simone. *The Coming of Age.* Translated by Patrick O'Brien. New York: Putnam, 1972.

de Beauvoir, Simone. *The Second Sex.* Translated by H.M. Parshley. New York: Knopf, Vintage Books, 1974.

Doyal, Lesley. *What Makes Women Sick: Gender and the Political Economy of Health.*
New Jersey: Rutgers University Press, 1995.

Ehrenreich, Barbara. *Complaints and Disorders: The Sexual Politics of Sickness.* New York: Old Westbury, 1973.

Eich, W., M. Hartman, A. Muller and H. Fischer. "The role of psychological factors in fibromyalgia syndrome." *Scan. J. Rheumatol. Supp.* 113 (2000): 30-31.

Estok, P. and R. O'Toole. "The Meanings of Menopause." *Health Care for Women International* 12 (1991): 27-39.

Finkler, Kaja. "A Theory of Life's Lesions: A Contribution to Solving the Mystery of Why Women Get Sick More Than Men." *Health Care for Women International* 21, no. 5 (2000): 433-455.

Frank, Arthur W. *The Wounded Storyteller: Body, Illness and Ethics.* Chicago and London: University of Chicago Press, 1995.

Frueh, Joanna. "Visible Difference: Women Artists and Aging." In *The Other Within Us: Feminist Explorations of Women and Aging,* edited by Marilyn Pearsall, 197-219. Colorado: Westview Press, 1997.

Goldberg, Burton. *Chronic Fatigue, Fibromyalgia and Environmental Illness.* Tiburon, CA: Future Medicine Publishers, 1998.

Gordon, L. *Heroes of Their Own Lives.* New York: Viking, 1988.

Gracely, R. H., F. Petzke, J. M. Wolf and D. J. Clairw. "Functional magnetic resonance imaging evidence of augmented pain processing in fibromyalgia." *Arthritis Rheumatology* 46, no. 5 (May 2002): 1333-1343.

Greer, Germaine. *The Change: Women, Aging and the Menopause.* Toronto: Random House, 1991.

Griner, Thomas. *What's Really Wrong With You? A Revolutionary Look At How Muscles Affect Your Health.* New York: Avery Publishing Group, 1996.

Groopman, J. "Hurting All Over." *The New Yorker*, November 13, 2000, 78-92.

Hadler, N. "Fibromylalgia: La maladie est morte. Vive la maladie." *Journal of Rheumatology* 25 (1998): 1250-1252.

Hadler, N. "If you have to prove you are ill, you can't get well." *Spine* 2 (1996): 2397-2400.

Hadler, N. "The Disabled, the Disallowed, the Disaffected and the Disavowed." *JOEM* 38, no. 3 (March 1996): 247-251.

Hart, B. and V. Grace. "Fatigue in Chronic Fatigue Syndrome: A Discourse Analysis of Women's Experiential Narratives." *Health Care for Women Intl.* 21, no. 3 (2000): 187-201.

Henderson, R. "Chronic fatigue syndrome an illness, court rules." (1998), http://www.edmontonjournal.com/news/alberta/042298ab2.html.

Henrikson, C., I. Gundmark, A. Bengtsson and A. Ek. "Living with Fibromyalgia Consequences for Everyday Life." *The Clinical Journal of Pain* 8, no. 2 (1992): 138-144.

Henriksson, C. and C. Burckhardt. "Impact of fibromyalgia on everyday life: a study of women in the USA and Sweden." *Disability Rehabilitation* 18, no. 5 (May 1996): 241-248.

Hiscock, M. "Complex reactions requiring empathy and knowledge: Psychological aspects of acute pain." *Professional Nurse* 12, (1994):158-160.

Holloway, Karla F. C. and Stephanie Demetrakopoulos. "Remembering Our Foremothers: Older Black Women, Politics of Age, Politics of Survival as Embodied in the Novels of Toni Morrison." In *The Other Within Us: Feminist Explorations of Women and Aging*, edited by Marilyn Pearsall, 177-195. Colorado: Westview Press, 1997.

Holmes, E. B. and L. M. Purdy. *Feminist Perspectives in Medical Ethics.* Bloomington: Indiana University Press, 1992.

Howard, Jennifer. "Getting Sensitive to Gender Sensitive Health Planning" *Canadian Women's Health Network* 3, no. 1/2 (Spring 2000). http://www.cwhn.ca/network-reseau/3-1/3-1pg7.html (accessed March 10, 2006).

Jackson, Marni. *Pain: the Fifth Vital Sign.* Canada: Random House, 2002.

Jensen, Karen. *Menopause: a Naturopathic Approach to the Transition Years.* Scarborough, Ont: Prentice Hall Canada, 1999.

Johnson Jackson, Jacquelyne. "The Plight of Older Black Women." In *The Other Within Us: Feminist Explorations of Women and Aging*, edited by Marilyn Pearsall, 37-42. Colorado: Westview Press, 1997.

Jones, John Verrier and Diana Ginn. "Fibromyalgia: The Canadian Courts Have Spoken." *Journal of the Canadian Rheumatology Association* (date unkown).

Keddy, Barbara A. "Women Living with Fibromyalgia: The Body/Mind Connection." Paper presented at the Women's Health Conference in Victoria, British Columbia, April 29, 2000.

Kerstin, Wentz, Lindberg, Lellemor and Hallberg. "Psychological Functioning in Women with Fibromyalgia: A Grounded Theory Study." *Health Care for Women International* 25, no. 8 (2004): 702-729.

Khalsa, Dharma Singh. *The Pain Cure.* New York: Time Warner Books, 1999.

Khraishi, Majed. "Evaluation of Fibromyalgia Syndrome." *Canadian Journal of CME* (February 2000): 111-119.

Landis, Carol. "Sleep Dysfunction and Fibromyalgia." In *Alternative Treatments for Fibromyalgia & Chronic Fatigue Syndrome*, edited by Mari Skelly and Andrea Helm, 209-211. California: Hunter House Publishers, 1999.

Landis, C. A., M. J. Lenta, J. Rothermel, S. C. Riffle, D. Chapman, D. Buchwald and J. L. Shaver. "Decreased Nocturnal Levels of Prolactin and Growth Hormone in Women with Fibromyalgia." *J. Clin. Endocrinol. Metab.* 86, no. 4 (April 2001):1672-1678.

Lorden, Lisa. "Obtaining Social Security Disability: How to Begin the Process." http://chronicfatigue.about.com/health/chronicfatigue/library/uc/uc_sdavisbegin.html (2000).

Lowe, J. C. "Thyroid status of 38 fibromyalgia patients: implications for the etiology of fibromyalgia." *Clinical Bull. Myofascial Ther.* 2, no. 1 (1997): 47-64.

MacWhannell, P. "Take the medical model out of menopause." *Nursing Times* 95, no. 41 (October 13, 1999): 45-46.

Maine, Margo. *Body Wars: Making Peace with Women's Bodies.* California: Gurze Books, 2000.

Makela, M. and M. Heliovaara. "Prevalence of fibromyalgia in the Finnish population."*British Medical Journal* 303 (1991): 216-219.

Malterud, K. "Understanding women in pain. New pathways suggested by Umea researchers: qualitative research and feminist perspectives." *Scandinavian Journal of Primary Health Care* 16, no. 4 (Dec. 1998):195-198.

Man, S. C., et al. *Questions and Answers about Fibromyalgia.* Winnipeg, MB: Henderson Books, 1998.

Martin, E. *The Woman in the Body: Cultural Analysis of Reproduction.* Boston: Beacon Press, 1987.

Martinez, J. E., M. B. Ferraz, A. M. Fontana and E. Atra. "Psychological aspects of Brazilian women with fibromyalgia." *Journal of Psychosomatic Research* 39, no. 2 (February 1995): 167-174.

Matsakis, A. *I Can't Get Over It: A Handbook For Trauma Survivors.* Oakland, CA: New Harbinger Publications, 1996.

McBeth, J. and A. J. Silman. "The role of psychiatric disorders in fibromyalgia." *Curr. Rheumatol. Rep.* 3, no. 2 (April 2001):157-164.

McCain, G., R. Cameron and J. Kennedy. "The Problem of Long-term Disability Payments and Litigation in Primary Fibromyalgia: The Canadian Perspective." *Journal of Rheumatology* 16, Supp. 19 (1989): 174-176.

McElmurry, B. J. and D. S. Huddleston. "Self-Care and Menopause: Critical Review of Research." *Health Care for Women International* 12 (1991): 15-23.

McGee, J. "Holistic Health and the Critique of Western Medicine." *Social Science and Medicine* 26, no. 8 (1988):775-784.

McSherry, J. "Fibromyalgia: Current Status," *Mature Medicine Canada*, (2000): 108-110.

Meisler, J. G. "Towards Optimal Health." *Journal of Women's Health* 8, no. 3 (1999): 313-320.
Mercer, C. "Cross-cultural attitudes to the menopause and the ageing female." *Age and Ageing* 28 (1999):12-17.

Mingo, C., J. Herman and M. A. Jasperse. "Women's Stories: Ethnic Variations in Women's Attitudes and Experiences of Menopause, Hysterectomy, and Hormone Replacement Therapy." *Journal of Women's Health and Gender-based Medicine* 9, no. 2 (2000): S27-S38.

Montero, L. and I. Hernandez. "Social functioning as a significant factor in women's help-seeking behaviour during the climacteric period." *Social Psychiatry and Psychiatric Epidemiology* 28 (1993): 178-183.

Moore Schaefer, K. "Struggling to maintain balance: A study of women living with fibromyalgia." *Journal of Advanced Nursing* 21, no. 11 (1995): 95-102.

Moore Schaefer, Karen. "Health patterns of women with fibromyalgia." *Journal of Advanced Nursing* 26, no. 3 (1997): 565-571.

Moss, P. "Negotiating Spaces in Home Environments: Older Women Living with Arthritis." *Social Science Medicine* 45, no.1 (1997): 23-33.

Neilson, W. R. and H. Merskey. "Psychological aspects of fibromyalgia." *Curr. Pain Headache Rep.* 5, no. 4 (August 2001):330-337.

Neumann, L. and D. Buskila. "Ethnocultural and educational differences in Israeli women correlate with pain perception in fibromyalgia." *Journal of Rheumatology* 25, no. 7 (July 1998): 1369-1373.

O'Leary Cobb, Janine. *Understanding Menopause.* Toronto: Key Porter Books, 1988.

O'Leary Cobb, Janine. "Reassuring the woman facing menopause: strategies and resources." *Patient Education and Counseling* 33 (1998): 281-287.

Palmer, P. "Pain and Possibilities." *Feminism and Psychology* 6, no. 3 (1996): 457-462.

Pasquali, Elaine Anne. "The Impact of Premature Menopause on Women's Experience of Self." *Journal of Holistic Nursing* 17, no. 4 (1999): 346-364.

Pellerino, Mark. *Fibromyalgia: Managing the Pain.* Ohio: Anaheim Publishing, 1997.

Picard, A. "Depression assistance hard to get in old age." *The Globe and Mail.* January 9, 2002.

Pirie, Marian. "Women and the Role of Illness: Rethinking Feminist Theory." *Canadian Review of Sociology and Anthropology* 25, no. 4 (1988): 628-648.

Potter, Joshua. "Physician Input Strengthens Claim: Helping Fibromyalgia Patients Obtain Social Security Benefits." *Journal of Musculoskeletal Medicine* 9, no. 9 (1992): 65-74.

Prescott, E., M. Kjoller, P. M. Bulow, B. Danneskiold-Samsoe and F. Kamper-Jorgensen. "Fibromyalgia in the adult Danish population: A Prevalence Study." *Scandinavian Journal of Rheumatology* 22 (1992): 233-237.

Price, K. and J. Cheek. "Exploring the nursing role in pain management from a post-structuralist perspective." *Journal of Advanced Nursing* 24 (1996): 890-898.

Radetsky, Peter. "The Gulf War Within." *Discovery* (August 1997): 69-75.

Raspe, H. and C. H. Baumgartner. "The epidemiology of the fibromyalgia syndrome in a German town." abstract, *Scandinavian Journal of Rheumatology*, Supp 94, no. 8 (1992): 15.

Richman, J. A., J. Flaherty and K. M. Rospenda. "Chronic Fatigue Syndrome: have flawed assumptions been derived from treatment—based studies?" *American Journal of Public Health* 84 (1994): 282-284.

Sack, J. and V. Payne. "Alberta Judge Denies Existence of Fibromyalgia." *Ontario Medical Review* (February 1995): 67-73.

Sahley, Billie Jay. *Malic Acid and Magnesium for Fibromyalgia and Chronic Pain Syndrome.* Texas: Pain and Stress Publications, 1966.

Scarry, Elaine. *The Body in Pain.* Oxford: Oxford University Press, 1985.

Schrager, C. "Questioning the Promise of Self-Help: A Reading of Women Who Love Too Much." *Feminist Studies* 19, no. 1 (Spring 1993): 176-192.

Sherman, J. J., D. C. Turk and A. Okifuji. *Clinical Journal of Pain* 16, no. 2 (June 2000): 127-134.

Simms, R. "Fibromyalgia Syndrome: Current Concepts in Pathophysiology, Clinical Features, and Management." *Arthritis Care and Research* 9, no. 4 (1996): 315-328.

Sirkin, Alicia. "Fibromyalgia Falls to Flowers: A Case History." *Alternative Medicine* 39 (January 2001): 76-85.

Skelly, Mari and Andrea Helm, eds. *Alternative Treatments for Fibromyalgia & Chronic Fatigue Syndrome.* California: Hunter House Publishers, 1999.

Soderberg, S., B. Lundman and J. Norberg. "Struggling for dignity: the meaning of women's experiences of living with fibromyalgia." *Qualitative Health Research* 9, no. 5 (September 1999): 575-587.

Sommer, B., N. Avis, P. Meyer, M. Ory, T. Madden, M. Kagawa-Singer, C. Mouton, N. O'Neill
Rasor and S. Adler. "Attitudes Toward Menopause and Aging Across Ethnic/Racial Groups." *Psychosomatic Medicine* 61 (1999): 868-875.

Starlanyl, Devin. *The Fibromyalgia Advocate.* Oakland: New Harbinger Publications, 1998.

Starlanyl, Devin and Mary Ellen Copeland. *Fibromyalgia & Chronic Myofascial Pain Syndrome.* Oakland: New Harbinger Publications, 1996.

Teitelbaum, Jacob. *From Fatigue to Fantastic.* Newsletter, Vol. 2, no.1 (June 1998).

Torpy, D. J., D. A. Papanicolaou, A. J. Lotsikas, R. L. Wilder, G. P. Chrousos and S. R. Pillemer. "Responses of the sympathetic nervous system and the hypothalamic-pituitary adrenal axis to interleukin-6: a pilot study in fibromyalgia." *Arthritis Rheumatology* 43, no. 4 (April 2000): 872-880.

Turk, Dennis. "Psychological Aspects of Chronic Pain." In *Alternative Treatments for Fibromyalgia & Chronic Fatigue Syndrome*, edited by Mari Skelly and Andrea Helm, 205-208. California: Hunter House Publishers, 1999.

Van Houdenhove, B. "Fibromyalgia: A challenge for modern medicine," *Clinical Rheumatology* 22 (2003):1–5.

Van Houdenhove, B., U. Egle, and P. Luyten. "The Role of Life Stress in Fibromyalgia," *Current Rheumatology Reports* 7 (2005): 365-370.

Wall, P. and R. Melzack. *The Challenge of Pain*. London: Penguin Science Books, 1996.

Wallace, D. and J. Wallace. *Fibromyalgia: An Essential Guide for Patients and Their Families*. New York: Oxford University Press, 2003.

Waxman, J. and S. M. Zatzkis. "Fibromyalgia and menopause: Examination of the Relationship." *Post Graduate Medicine* 80, no. 4 (September 15, 1986):165-171.

Welner, S. "Menopausal Issues." *Sexuality and Disability* 17, no. 3 (1999): 259-267.

Wentz, K. A., C. Lindberg, and L. R. Hallberg. "Psychological functioning in women with fibromyalgia: a grounded theory study," *Health Care for Women International* 25, no. 8 (September 2004): 702–729.

White, K. and M. Harth. "The Fibromyalgia Problem: Comment" *Journal of Rheumatology* 25, no. 5 (May 1998): 1022-1023.

Wilkinson, R. "A Non-pharmacological approach to pain relief." *Professional Nurse* 11, no. 4 (1996): 222-224.

Williamson, Miryam Ehrlich. *Fibromyalgia: a Comprehensive Approach.* New York: Walker & Co., 1996.

Winterich, J. and D. Umberson. "How Women Experience Menopause: The Importance of Social Context." *Journal of Women and Aging* 11, no. 4 (1999): 57-73.

Wolfe, F. "The Fibromyalgia Problem." *The Journal of Rheumatology* 24, no. 7 (1997): 1247-1249.

Wolfe, F., K. Ross, J. Anderson, I. J. Russell and L. Herbert. "The prevalence and characteristics of fibromyalgia in the general population." *Arthritis Rheumatology* 38 (1995): 19-28.

Yunus, M. B., M. A. Khan, K. K. Rawlings, J. R. Green, J. M. Olson and S. Shah.
"Genetic linkage analysis of multicase families with fibromyalgia syndrome." *Journal of Rheumatology* 26, no. 2 (February 1999): 408-412.

World Health Organization. *The international classification of impairments, disabilities, and handicaps.* New York: W H O, 1980.

978-0-595-44371-0
0-595-44371-0

Printed in the United States
104464LV00002B/12/A

9 780595 443710